OSCEs, EMQs and
BOFs in Obstetrics and Gynaecology

Second Edition

To Roger and Ammy, our support systems

For Elsevier
Commissioning Editor: Pauline Graham
Development Editor: Helen Leng
Project Manager: Elouise Ball
Design Direction: Erik Bigland
Illustrator: Richard Morris
Illustration Manager: Merlyn Harvey

OSCEs, EMQs and BOFs in Obstetrics and Gynaecology

Second Edition

Janice Rymer MD FRCOG FRANZCOG

Professor of Obstetrics and Gynaecology
Kings College School of Medicine at Guy's and St Thomas' Hospitals
London, UK

Hasib Ahmed FRCOG

Consultant in Obstetrics and Gynaecology
Medway Maritime Hospital, Gillingham
Kent, UK

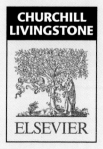

CHURCHILL LIVINGSTONE

ELSEVIER

Edinburgh London New York Oxford Philadelphia St Louis Sydney Toronto 2008

CHURCHILL
LIVINGSTONE
ELSEVIER

CHURCHILL LIVINGSTONE
An imprint of Elsevier Limited

First edition 1998
Second edition 2008

ISBN-13: 9780443103193

British Library Cataloguing in Publication Data
A catalogue record for this book is available from the British Library

Library of Congress Cataloging in Publication Data
A catalog record for this book is available from the Library of Congress

Note
Knowledge and best practice in this field are constantly changing. As new research and experience broaden our knowledge, changes in practice, treatment and drug therapy may become necessary or appropriate. Readers are advised to check the most current information provided (i) on procedures featured or (ii) by the manufacturer of each product to be administered, to verify the recommended dose or formula, the method and duration of administration, and contraindications. It is the responsibility of the practitioner, relying on their own experience and knowledge of the patient, to make diagnoses, to determine dosages and the best treatment for each individual patient, and to take all appropriate safety precautions. To the fullest extent of the law, neither the publisher nor the authors assume any liability for any injury and/or damage to persons or property arising out of or related to any use of the material contained in this book.

The Publisher

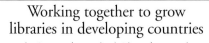

Working together to grow
libraries in developing countries

www.elsevier.com | www.bookaid.org | www.sabre.org

ELSEVIER   BOOK AID International   Sabre Foundation

Printed in China

Preface

Our previous textbook concentrated on the Objective Structured Clinical Examinations (OSCEs) in Obstetrics and Gynaecology and we had extensive coverage of topics in obstetric, gynaecology, contraception, neonatal medicine, and sexually transmitted diseases. Since the first edition there have been significant changes to the format of undergraduate and postgraduate examinations in obstetrics and gynaecology. In line with these changes the exciting new edition includes the new format Extended Matching Questions (EMQs) and Best of Fives (BOFs). The new formats are deemed more robust at assessing knowledge by reducing ambiguity. The informed candidate is guided to the most likely answer and the chance of success by random choice is reduced. By adding in these different formats, we hope now to provide the undergraduate and postgraduate with revision material for both the clinical and written examinations.

First and foremost we thank all the patients for volunteering to be photographed. Special thanks to the Medical Illustration Department of Guy's and St Thomas' Hospitals and the Departments of Histopathology and Antenatal Ultrasound at Medway Maritime Hospital. We also thank Dr Toh Lick Tan, Dr Eduard Cortes, Dr Hossam Hamid and Mr Ahmad Sayesneh for advice on some of the questions. Finally, we thank Tanya Ravlen for typing the manuscript.

Contents

Introduction to OSCEs

Objective structured clinical examination (OSCEs) as a method of student assessment are well established and are gradually being introduced into postgraduate assessment. OSCEs have been developed because they are valid, reliable, have high fidelity and are a feasible method of assessment.

Depending on the particular examination there are a varying number of stations. At each station the candidate has to perform a task, and these stations may be testing knowledge, skills, communication or problem-solving ability or a combination of any of these. Depending on the type of station, there may be a role player, a patient, a photograph, a pelvic model or a clinical scenario.

At each station you have a defined period of time at the end of which a bell or buzzer sounds and you move on, usually in a clockwise direction, to the next station. Within the OSCE circuit there may be rest stations and these stations often provide information to prepare you for the following station.

Within this book we have arranged four typical OSCE circuits. Each of these circuits consists of 20 stations. As it is impossible to be interactive in a book, we have organised the structured orals and communication stations separately. Normally within an OSCE circuit the interactive and the structured oral stations would be intermingled with the other stations.

Knowledge or factual stations

These stations are purely assessing your knowledge regarding certain subjects. The material provided may be a photograph, results of investigations or a clinical scenario. Within the four following circuits there are many examples of these. When performing an OSCE, be certain to listen carefully to the examiner's instructions as to where to write on your answer sheet.

Clinical skills stations

At these stations there may well be patients on whom you are asked to perform a skill. With regard to pelvic examinations, it is unlikely that there will be live patients and more commonly you would be asked to do a speculum examination or bimanual examination on a plastic model. If you are put into the situation of examining a plastic model, it would be appropriate to talk to the model as if it were a live patient to show that you are quite accustomed to this scenario.

Summary

An OSCE ensures that each candidate is exposed to the same examination questions and environment. Therefore the marking is very rigid and standardised.

Objective structured clinical examination (OSCEs)

Circuit **A**

1.1 Look at the photograph and state three differential diagnoses.

1.2 What three symptoms may she have presented with?

1.3 Name three appropriate investigations.

1.4 What corrective procedure should she have?

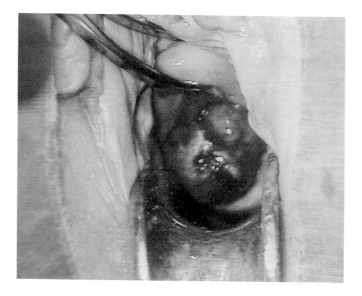

2.1 The baby in the photograph is 2 days old. What treatment is he receiving?

2.2 Name the condition that is being treated.

2.3 In this case the cause was physiological. Describe the mechanisms of jaundice. Specify three points.

2.4 How is unconjugated bilirubin transported in the serum?

2.5 Describe two clinical features of kernicterus other than jaundice.

2.6 Name two potential long-term sequelae of kernicterus.

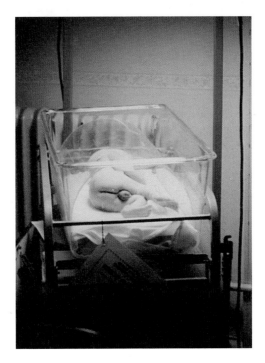

3.1   What are these pills used for?

3.2   What do these pills (excluding the larger pills) contain?

3.3   Apart from the obvious benefit of this medication, name four other benefits.

3.4   If a woman missed the first two pills in the red section, what would you advise her to do?

3.5   Name two absolute contraindications to this preparation.

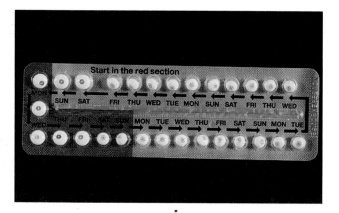

A woman (para 2 gravida 3) presented at 33 weeks with vaginal bleeding. Her ultrasound scan (USS) is illustrated. (Her first delivery was by lower segment caesarean section (LSCS), and her second was a normal delivery.) Her blood group is O rhesus positive.

4.1 What is the cause of her bleeding?

4.2 What would you have found on abdominal examination? Name two features.

4.3 What would your management of this woman be? Name two aspects.

4.4 How would you deliver her?

4.5 If the placenta was anterior, would anything concern you?

4.6 Name three other causes of antepartum haemorrhage (APH) at 33 weeks.

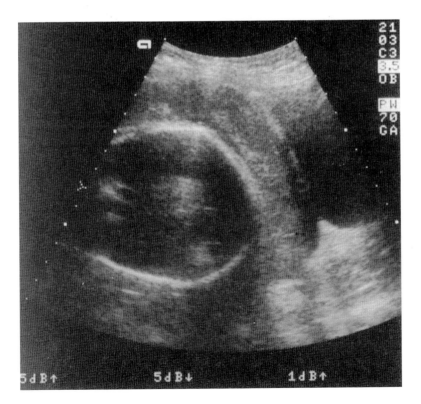

Ms JJ has had a quadrivalent screening test performed in this pregnancy. The result is shown.

5.1   Which four parameters have been measured? (No abbreviations)

5.2   In the results what does MoM stand for?

5.3   What is the usual risk cutoff which defines a positive screening test result?

5.4   Name the most appropriate diagnostic test which Ms JJ should be counselled for.

5.5   Name a reliable first trimester screening test for chromosomal abnormalities.

5.6   At which gestation should this be performed in order to calculate a numerical risk?

DOWN'S SYNDROME AND NEURAL TUBE DEFECT SCREENING   **Report dated 18 Apr 06**

Surname	:	
Forename(s)	:	
Hospital no.	:	
Date of birth	:	
LMP	:	23/12/05
Date of sample	:	11/04/06
Date received	:	13/04/06
Doctor	:	

CLINICAL DETAILS AND TEST RESULTS

DEPM code	:			
Previous NTD	:	None		
Previous Down's	:	None		
Insulin-dependent diabetes	:	None		
Maternal age at EDD	:	29 years		
Scan measure	:	BPD		
Gestation at date of sample	:	15 weeks 4 days (by dates)		
		15 weeks 4 days (by BPD scan)		
Gestation used	:	Scan estimate (BPD)		
Weight	:	76.0 kg		
Ethnic origin	:	Caucasian		
MS-AFP level	:	11.50 Iu/ml	:	0.49 MoM
UE3 level	:	2.40 nmol/l	:	0.83 MoM
Free beta-hCG level	:	38.39 ng/ml	:	2.56 MoM
Inhibin-A level	:	180.10 pg/ml	:	1.24 MoM

INTERPRETATION

Screening result	:	***SCREEN POSITIVE***
Reason	:	Increased risk of Down's syndrome
Risk of Down's	:	1 in 90 (at term)

* A screen positive result indicates an increased risk of having a pregnancy with Down's syndrome or a neural tube defect. Most women with screen positive results will not have an affected pregnancy

A 24-year-old primigravida presents at 32 weeks with a history of a large loss of clear fluid from the vagina.

6.1 How would you confirm the diagnosis of premature rupture of membranes (PROM)?

6.2 What is the differential diagnosis? Name two conditions.

6.3 What investigations would you perform? Name three.

6.4 What drug treatment might you consider and why? Name three classes of drug.

6.5 What is the percentage chance of spontaneous labour within the next 10 days?

A woman presents to the gynaecology clinic with an offensive vaginal discharge. The speculum examination shown below is performed.

7.1   Describe what you see.

7.2   You take a high vaginal sample, mix it with a drop of saline and look at it under the microscope. You see a flagellate parasite. What is the diagnosis?

7.3   Where else (apart from the vagina) would you find this organism?

7.4   How is this organism acquired?

7.5   What other organism is often found in association with it?

7.6   Name three aspects of your management.

7.7   What follow-up would you arrange?

7.8   What is the commonest cause of vaginal discharge?

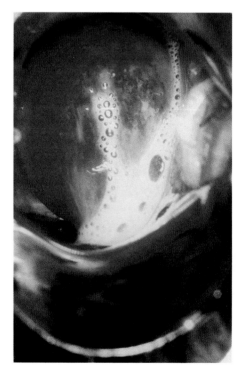

8.1   What abnormality do you see in the illustration?

8.2   What is the 'group' of abnormalities called?

8.3   What other group of abnormalities would this alert you to?

8.4   What symptoms may this woman present with? Name two.

8.5   If this woman were to become pregnant, what problems may she encounter in labour? Name two.

8.6   Name two structures of which the paramesonephric ducts are precursors?

8.7   What does the lower third of the vagina develop from?

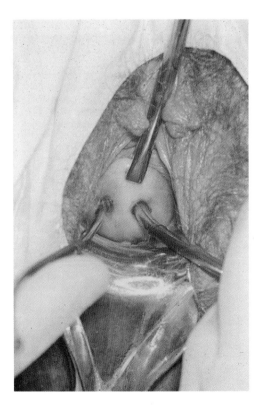

Look at the photograph.

9.1   Regarding the report shown, name the five classification groups of maternal deaths.

9.2   In the report, what were the three commonest causes for direct maternal deaths (in the correct order)?

9.3   In a pregnant woman with a history of previous deep vein thrombosis in pregnancy and no other risk factors, what are the RCOG recommendations for treatment? State medication, when to start and duration of therapy.

9.4   In a higher risk woman (multiple thromboembolic events in pregnancy), what are the recommendations?

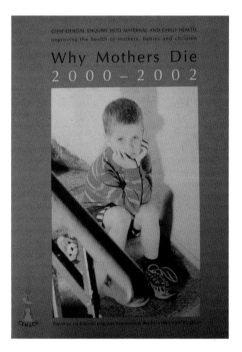

A 38-year-old primigravid woman has been admitted at 33 weeks gestation. She booked with a blood pressure (BP) of 110/60 mmHg. She has 2+ proteinuria and her BP is consistently 175/105 mmHg. She is complaining of visual disturbances.

10.1 What abnormalities are revealed in the haematology result? Name two.

10.2 Name two further maternal investigations you would arrange.

10.3 Name three principal risks for the woman and her fetus that would concern you.

10.4 She develops abdominal pain. What are the two most likely causes?

10.5 Her BP that afternoon goes up to 175/110. What antihypertensive would you give her in the first instance (and state the correct dose)?

Guy's Hospital **Department of Haematology**		Surname	A
		Forename	F
Date 10.9.06		Sex	F
		DOB	30.9.70
		Number	660435
Haemoglobin	13.4 g/dl		
White cell count	$9.3 \times 10^9/l$		
Platelet count	$94 \times 10^{12}/l$		
PCV	0.45		
MCV	83 fl		
MCHC	29 g/dl		

Miss SE is 19 years old and is in her first pregnancy. Her last menstrual period was approximately 2 months ago and was normal. Her GP has carried out a pregnancy test, which was positive, and has sent her for a transvaginal ultrasound scan. He is concerned because Miss SE has been complaining of pain and tenderness in the right iliac fossa. A photograph of the ultrasound findings is shown.

11.1 Describe the appearance of the uterine cavity. Name two features.

11.2 What organs giving rise to A and B are seen adjacent to the uterus?

11.3 What must be visualised during real-time ultrasound scanning to confirm that the fetus is alive?

11.4 What is the likely aetiology of B?

11.5 What is the usual outcome of B?

11.6 What two complications may occur with B and result in abdominal pain?

11.7 What is the function of B?

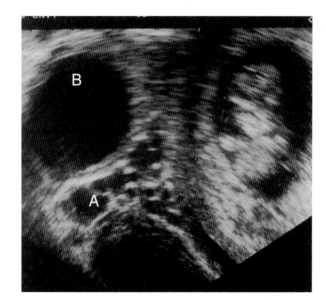

Mrs PP gave birth to a live baby boy 2 weeks ago. The midwife looking after her is worried because Mrs PP is not showing much interest in her newborn son. She spends a lot of the day in bed and is tearful.

12.1 What is the likely diagnosis?

12.2 Name three features which would confirm your diagnosis.

12.3 How common is the problem?

12.4 List three risk factors for postnatal depression.

12.5 Name two types of drugs that may be prescribed for Mrs PP.

13.1 Name the four hormones.

13.2 What two types of cells are involved in the synthesis of C?

13.3 What cells produce D?

13.4 What effect does D have on cervical mucus?

13.5 What hormone causes the temperature rise illustrated?

13.6 At birth, how many oocytes are present?

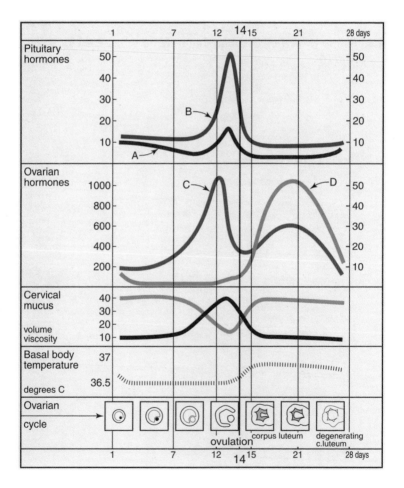

A 30-year-old, para 2 gravida 2 woman presents to the gynaecology clinic saying that she has premenstrual syndrome (PMS).

14.1 What is the commonest reported psychological symptom of PMS?

14.2 What are the two most common physical symptoms of PMS?

14.3 How do you make the diagnosis?

14.4 What relieves PMS physiologically?

14.5 Name five treatments.

The illustrated USS is from a 74-year-old woman.

15.1 Describe the scan. Name three features.

15.2 What is the most likely diagnosis?

15.3 What operation would be performed?

15.4 Name two symptoms she may have presented with.

15.5 What three methods may be used to screen for this disease?

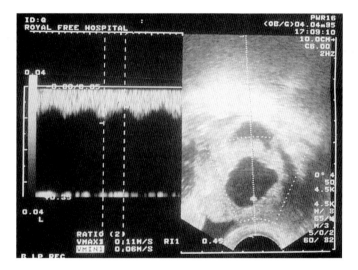

This 74-year-old presented with a 'lump' down below.

16.1 What is the diagnosis?

16.2 What is the main predisposing factor?

16.3 What conservative therapy could be instituted?

16.4 What surgical therapy could be offered?

16.5 Why might this present postmenopausally?

16.6 If she presented 2 years later with vault prolapse, what surgical operations could you offer? Name two.

16.7 In the outpatient department, what instrument would you use to examine this woman?

16.8 Name two conditions that may aggravate this condition.

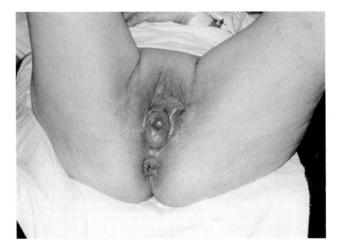

17.1 What two abnormalities does the X-ray show?

17.2 Name three symptoms she may have.

17.3 What other investigations would you order? Name three.

17.4 What is the probable diagnosis?

17.5 Name one treatment.

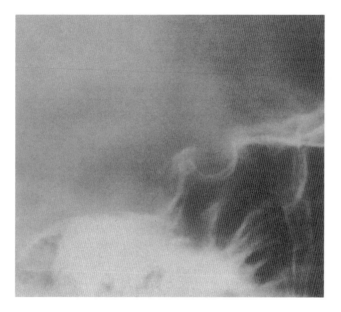

18.1 Name the three types of breech illustrated.

18.2 Name two maternal causes.

18.3 Name two fetal causes.

18.4 What investigation would you perform in a primigravida at 37 weeks with a breech presentation if you were contemplating a vaginal delivery?

18.5 At term, what is the incidence of breech presentation?

18.6 What procedure would you offer at term?

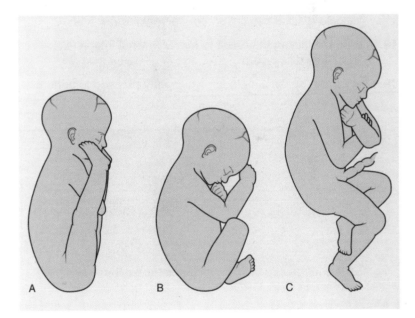

Mrs MR is 39 years old and has two children aged 14 and 11 who are alive and well. She is now 18 weeks pregnant and had an amniocentesis 2 weeks ago. The result is shown.

19.1   What is the risk of miscarriage associated with an amniocentesis procedure?

19.2   List four other complications that have been described following amniocentesis.

19.3   What is an alternative procedure to amniocentesis which yields a quicker cell culture for karyotyping?

19.4   After explaining the result to Mrs MR, what intervention should be discussed?

19.5   List three medical methods which may be used to perform this intervention.

Guy's Hospital
Department of Cytogenetics

Date 8.3.06

Surname	R
Forename	M
Sex	F
DOB	22.10.67
Number	S70719

Karyotype Report

Sample   Amniotic fluid

Cell culture   +ve

Karyotype   47   XY

Male fetus with trisomy 21

Suggest review by Obstetrician ASAP

A measurement is being performed on the woman shown below.

20.1 What are the causes of large for dates? Name five.

20.2 Name three investigations you would perform.

20.3 What is the measurement called?

20.4 What is its relevance?

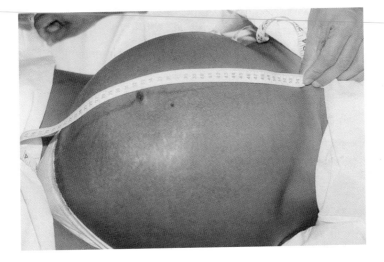

1.1   Cervical carcinoma, cervical polyp, endometrial polyp/ pedunculated fibroid [Marks 3]

1.2   Postcoital bleeding, intermenstrual bleeding, menorrhagia [Marks 3]

1.3   TVS, cervical smear, endometrial biopsy, hysteroscopy, biopsy of lesion [Marks 3]

1.4   Removal of polyp, excision biopsy of lesion [Marks 1]

2.1   Phototherapy [Marks 1]

2.2   Jaundice (raised serum bilirubin) [Marks 1]

2.3   Raised neonatal PCV, immature liver, poor conjugation, dehydration, raised unconjugated bilirubin [Marks 3]

2.4   Bound to albumin [Marks 1]

2.5   Poor feeding, drowsiness, opisthotonos, convulsions [Marks 2]

2.6   Residual brain damage, choreoathetosis, mental retardation [Marks 2]

3.1   Contraception [Marks 1]

3.2   Oestrogen, progestogen [Marks 2]

3.3   Cycle control, less bleeding, less pain, protects against ovarian cancer, protects against endometrial cancer, prevents bone loss, alleviates symptoms of endometriosis, acne improvement, protects against PID [Marks 4]

3.4   Nothing [Marks 1]

3.5   Past history of DVT, past history of CVA, focal migraine, gross obesity, >40 cigarettes/day, high blood pressure, severe diabetes [Marks 2]

4.1 Placenta praevia [Marks 1]

4.2 Soft uterus, presenting part high [Marks 2]

4.3 Keep in hospital, always have blood available/group and cross-match, IV (intravenous) line [Marks 2]

4.4 LSCS [Marks 1]

4.5 The possibility of morbid adherence of the placenta requiring hysterectomy [Marks 1]

4.6 Abruption, marginal edge bleed, vasa praevia, local causes [Marks 3]

5.1 (Maternal) serum alphafetoprotein, oestriol, beta human chorionic gonadotrophin, inhibin A [Marks 4]

5.2 Multiples of the Median [Marks 1]

5.3 1:250 or 1:300 (accept either) [Marks 1]

5.4 Amniocentesis [Marks 1]

5.5 Nuchal translucency scan [Marks 1]

5.6 11 weeks and 5 days to 13 weeks and 5 days gestation [Marks 2]

6.1 Speculum examination and see pooling of liquor in the vagina [Marks 1]

6.2 Urinary incontinence, vaginal discharge [Marks 2]

6.3 Endocervical swab, white blood count (WBC), ultrasound scan, fibronectin swab, C-reactive (CR) protein, mid-stream urine (MSU) [Marks 3]

6.4 Tocolytics if contracting, steroids for lung maturation, antibiotics for prophylaxis [Marks 3]

6.5 >90% [Marks 1]

7.1 A frothy yellowy white discharge [Marks 1]

7.2 *Trichomonas vaginalis* [Marks 1]

7.3 Urethra, upper genital tract/endocervix [Marks 1]

7.4 Sexually [Marks 1]

7.5 Gonococcus [Marks 1]

7.6 Metronidazole, screen for other sexually transmitted diseases, advise barrier contraception until disease resolves, screen and treat the partner/partners [Marks 3]

7.7 Repeat swabs after treatment [Marks 1]

7.8 Candida [Marks 1]

8.1 Two cervices [Marks 1]

8.2 Müllerian duct abnormalities [Marks 1]

8.3 Renal tract abnormalities [Marks 1]

8.4 Recurrent miscarriage, infertility, menorrhagia [Marks 2]

8.5 Incoordinate uterine action, malpresentations, retained placenta [Marks 2]

8.6 Fallopian tubes, uterus, upper two-thirds of the vagina [Marks 2]

8.7 Urogenital sinus [Marks 1]

9.1 Direct, indirect, coincidental (fortuitous), late, pregnancy related [Marks 3]

9.2 Thrombosis/thromboembolism, haemorrhage, hypertensive disorders of pregnancy [Marks 3]

9.3 Low molecular weight heparin (LMWH), start after delivery, continue for up to 6 weeks [Marks 3]

9.4 LMW heparin throughout pregnancy and six weeks postpartum [Marks 1]

Station 10   ANSWERS   Circuit A

10.1 Haemoconcentration/high haemoglobin/high packed cell volume (PCV), low platelets [Marks 2]

10.2 24-hour urinalysis for protein, liver function tests, MSU, clotting studies, serum urea and electrolytes (U&E), urate [Marks 2]

10.3 Eclampsia, abruption causing fetal distress, death, disseminated intravascular coagulation (DIC), cerebrovascular accident [Marks 3]

10.4 Liver tenderness – subcapsular haemorrhages, placental abruption [Marks 2]

10.5 Hydrallazine (initially in a 5-mg i.v. bolus), nifedipine (10 mg sublingually) [Marks 1]

Station 11   ANSWERS   Circuit A

11.1 Intrauterine gestation sac, identifiable fetus within the gestation sac [Marks 2]

11.2 A – Bowel, B – Ovary [Marks 2]

11.3 Fetal heart movement [Marks 1]

11.4 Corpus luteum cyst of pregnancy [Marks 1]

11.5 Spontaneous resolution by the end of the first trimester [Marks 1]

11.6 Cyst haemorrhage/(rupture), cyst/ovarian torsion [Marks 2]

11.7 Steroid hormone secretion in first trimester/oestrogen progestogen secretion in first trimester [Marks 1]

Station 12   ANSWERS   Circuit A

12.1 Postnatal depression [Marks 1]

12.2 Insomnia, loss of appetite, irritability, inability to cope, self-reproach [Marks 3]

12.3 Approximately 25% of new mothers (20–30%) [Marks 1]

12.4 Depression in index pregnancy, age >30, history of depression/ previous postnatal depression, history of severe pre-menstrual syndrome, poor socioeconomic support, traumatic pregnancy/ delivery, poor neonatal outcome [Marks 3]

12.5 Oestrogens, progestogens, antidepressants [Marks 2]

Station 13	ANSWERS	Circuit **A**

13.1 A – FSH, B – LH, C – Oestradiol, D – Progesterone [Marks 4]

13.2 Theca cells of the stroma, granulosa cells of the follicle [Marks 2]

13.3 Luteinised granulosa cells of the corpus luteum [Marks 1]

13.4 It makes mucus hostile or impenetrable to sperm [Marks 1]

13.5 Progesterone [Marks 1]

13.6 2 million (1–4 million) [Marks 1]

Station 14	ANSWERS	Circuit **A**

14.1 Irritability [Marks 1]

14.2 Abdominal bloating, breast tenderness [Marks 2]

14.3 Menstrual symptom diary [Marks 1]

14.4 Onset of menstruation [Marks 1]

14.5 Explanation and reassurance, relaxation techniques, combined oral contraception (COC)/hormone, replacement therapy (HRT), nonsteroidal anti-inflammatory drugs (NSAIDs), pyridoxine, bromocriptine, evening primrose oil, diuretics, selective serotonin reuptake inhibitors (SSRIs) [Marks 5]

Station 15	ANSWERS	Circuit **A**

15.1 Cystic structure, solid elements, smooth capsule, free fluid [Marks 3]

15.2 Ovarian carcinoma [Marks 1]

15.3 Staging laparotomy, TAH and BSO and omentectomy [Marks 1]

15.4 Abdominal distention, pressure effects on other organs, problems in micturation/defaecation, pelvic pain/abdominal pain [Marks 2]

15.5 Tumour markers, vaginal ultrasound, vaginal examination, Doppler bloodflow [Marks 3]

Station 16	ANSWERS	Circuit A

16.1 Uterovaginal prolapse/procidentia [Marks 1]

16.2 Childbirth [Marks 1]

16.3 Ring pessary/shelf pessary [Marks 1]

16.4 Vaginal hysterectomy, anterior and posterior repair [Marks 1]

16.5 Lack of oestrogen [Marks 1]

16.6 Le Forts procedure, sacrospinous fixation, sacrocolpopexy, Moscowitz procedure [Marks 2]

16.7 Sim's speculum [Marks 1]

16.8 Chronic cough, constipation, pelvic mass, obesity [Marks 2]

Station 17	ANSWERS	Circuit A

17.1 Double flooring of the pituitary fossa, enlargement of the pituitary fossa [Marks 2]

17.2 Galactorrhoea, amenorrhoea, visual symptoms, headaches, infertility [Marks 3]

17.3 Serum prolactin, visual fields mapping, thyroid function tests, MRI/CT of the pituitary fossa [Marks 3]

17.4 Pituitary adenoma [Marks 1]

17.5 Bromocriptine/carbergoline, hypophysectomy, radiation therapy [Marks 1]

18.1 A – Extended/frank, B – Flexed, C – Footling [Marks 3]

18.2 Grand multiparity, uterine anomalies, pelvic tumour, bony pelvic abnormality [Marks 2]

18.3 Fetal abnormality, extended neck, multiple gestation, prematurity [Marks 2]

18.4 USS [Marks 1]

18.5 Less than 5% [Marks 1]

18.6 External cephalic version [Marks 1]

19.1 1:100 [Marks 1]

19.2 Oligohydramnios, amniotic bands, talipes, congenital dislocation of the hip, rhesus isoimmunisation, neonatal respiratory distress syndrome (RDS), antepartum haemorrhage [Marks 4]

19.3 Chorionic villus sampling/biopsy [Marks 1]

19.4 Termination of pregnancy [Marks 1]

19.5 Intra-amniotic prostaglandin $F_2\alpha$, extra-amniotic prostaglandin E_2, vaginal prostaglandin analogue/gemeprost [Marks 3]

20.1 Maternal obesity, adnexal pathology, uterine fibroids, multiple pregnancy, fetal abnormality, macrosomic fetus, hydropic fetus, polyhydramnios [Marks 5]

20.2 USS, glucose tolerance test, antibodies (to check for isoimmunisation) [Marks 3]

20.3 Symphysiofundal height [Marks 1]

20.4 One centimetre corresponds to 1 week of gestation. (It is more useful if performed by the same examiner each time) [Marks 1]

Objective structured clinical examination (OSCEs)

Circuit B

Mrs PP had a **Ventouse extraction 4 days ago**. She had experienced spontaneous rupture of membranes 20 hours prior to augmentation with Syntocinon. The total length of her labour was 16 hours and the placenta was noted to be irregular in one area. She is feeling feverish with cramping abdominal pain. Her observation chart is shown.

1.1 Describe three abnormal features shown on her chart.

1.2 The lochia is offensive. On examination, the uterus is 16 weeks size and tender with a patulous cervical os. What is your working diagnosis? Name two features.

1.3 List three investigations you would arrange.

1.4 In general terms, what medical treatment would you start?

1.5 Which operative procedure may be necessary?

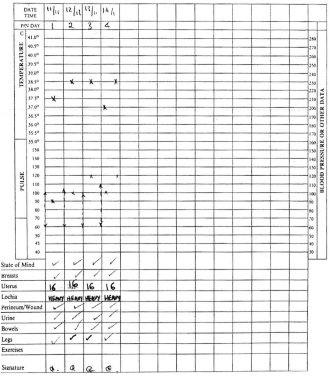

POST NATAL RECORD

Mrs MG is in the ninth week of her pregnancy. She has experienced severe nausea and vomiting over the last 3 weeks and light vaginal bleeding over the last 24 hours. A transvaginal ultrasound scan has been performed and a photograph of the findings is shown.

2.1   Describe the appearances of the uterine cavity (two features).

2.2   From the appearance of the scan, what is the likely placentation?

2.3   Two active fetal hearts are seen and the cervix is closed. What is the diagnosis?

2.4   Which two factors contribute to anaemia in this pregnancy?

2.5   Name two factors which predispose to multiple pregnancy.

2.6   Can the zygosity be predicted from the USS findings?

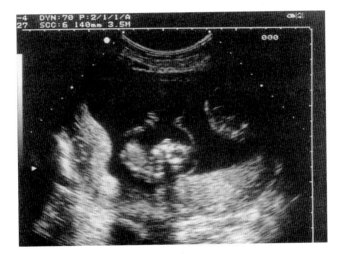

3.1 In the photograph, which structure in the neonatal skull is being examined?

3.2 Which pairs of bones form the boundaries of this structure? Name two.

3.3 If the skin over this structure is sunken, what should you suspect?

3.4 If the skin over this structure is very tense, what does this suggest?

3.5 At what age does this structure usually close?

3.6 What is the term given to a subperiosteal haematoma of the neonatal skull?

3.7 What clinical feature is pathognomonic of this?

3.8 List two complications of the above condition (Q. 3.6).

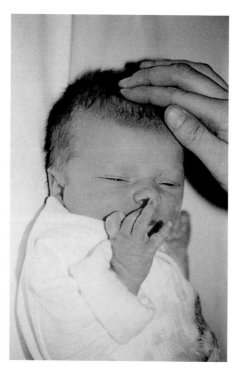

4.1   Name the two intrauterine contraceptive devices (IUCDs) illustrated.

4.2   Name two ways that these may provide contraception.

4.3   When should each of these be changed?

4.4   Name two complications of their use.

4.5   Name two absolute contraindications to the device on the right.

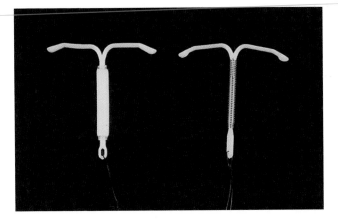

5.1   What organisms are seen on the smear?

5.2   What is the diagnosis?

5.3   Name two common symptoms of this condition.

5.4   On speculum examination, what would you expect to see?

5.5   Name three swabs you would take.

5.6   Name two treatments.

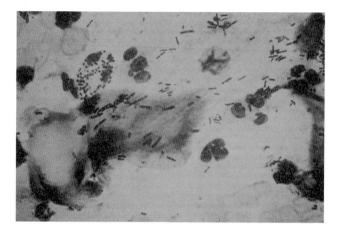

6.1   Define perinatal mortality rate (PNMR).

6.2   What is the national PNMR in the UK?

6.3   What are the major determinants of perinatal mortality?
Specify three.

6.4   At what maternal age is the perinatal mortality rate at its lowest?

6.5   A report of a regular confidential enquiry is shown in the
photograph. Which areas of the UK contribute to this report?

6.6   For the purposes of this report, what is the lower limit of the
birthweight of babies included in the intrapartum-related deaths?

6.7   After exclusion of babies with gross life-threatening abnormalities,
which deaths in terms of timing are included in the intrapartum
death group?

Confidential Enquiry into Maternal and Child Health

PERINATAL MORTALITY
SURVEILLANCE REPORT 2004

England, Wales and Northern Ireland

March 2006

CEMACH

Mrs Smith is a 24-year-old woman who has reached 30 weeks gestation in her first pregnancy. Her BP was 100/65 mmHg at booking. She now has a BP of 150/95 mmHg and 3+ proteinuria. Her biochemistry is illustrated.

7.1   What specific symptoms would you ask her about? Name two.

7.2   Name three clinical signs you would look for.

7.3   What abnormal result is displayed in the biochemistry?

7.4   Where would you manage this patient?

7.5   What fetal investigations would you do? Name two.

7.6   What are the chances of this condition recurring in the next pregnancy?

Department of Clinical Chemistry St. Elsewheres NHS Trust

Surname Smith	**First Name** Mary	**D.O.B** 27.03.82	**Hosp No** 123216
Consult Rymer	**Ward** Antenatal	**Report Date**	21.07.06

			n.r.
Sodium	135	mmol/l	(135–145)
Potassium	4.3	mmol/l	(3.5–5.0)
Urea	4.9	mmol/l	(2.5–7.5)
Creatinine	90	μmol/l	(65–101)
Alk. phosphatase	209	U/l	(38–126)
Albumin	35	g/l	(35–47)
Total protein	65	g/l	(64–80)
Alan. transaminase	20	U/l	(<55)
Total bilirubin	5	μmol/l	(<22)
Urate	0.40	mmol/l	(0.16–0.36)

A 35-year-old primigravida presented to the labour ward at 38 weeks gestation with constant abdominal pain, some vaginal bleeding and an irritable uterus. Her BP was 160/100 mmHg. Her FBC is shown.

8.1 What is the probable diagnosis?

8.2 What other investigations are important in the immediate management of this case? Name three.

8.3 On examination, what would the uterus feel like?

8.4 What management would you institute for the mother? Name three aspects.

8.5 If the CTG showed late decelerations in response to the uterine activity, what would you do?

8.6 With these cases, if maternal death occurs, what is the most likely cause?

Guy's Hospital **Department of Haematology**		Surname	J
		Forename	J
Date 21.10.06		Sex	F
		DOB	23.7.71
		Number	124215
Haemoglobin	12.4 g/dl		
White cell count	12.4×10^9/l		
Platelets	60×10^{12}/l		
PVC	0.42		
MCV	88 fl		

This woman presented with oligomenorrhoea.

9.1 What other symptom did she present with?

9.2 What is the likely diagnosis?

9.3 Name two hormone levels that are raised in this condition.

9.4 What serum protein is reduced?

9.5 What management would you advise, assuming she did not want to conceive? Name two aspects.

9.6 In later life, what may she be at risk of? Name one condition.

9.7 Name two histological features of the ovary.

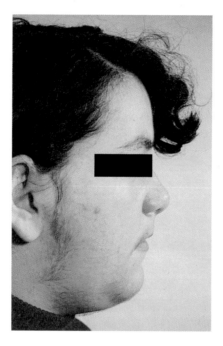

10.1 What classic symptoms may this woman have presented with? Name two.

10.2 As her GP, what would you do after receiving this report?

10.3 If the diagnosis is confirmed and is stage 1b, what is the appropriate treatment?

10.4 Name four risk factors for this disease.

10.5 What is the 5-year survival for stage 1 disease?

10.6 What age group has the highest incidence of this disease?

Mrs VH, age 66, had a vaginal hysterectomy 3 days ago. Her postoperative observation chart is shown.

11.1 What abnormalities can you identify? Specify two.

11.2 List four routine examinations you would perform.

11.3 List two microbiological investigations you would arrange.

11.4 Vaginal examination reveals marked tenderness of the vault. A transvaginal ultrasound report demonstrated a 7 cm × 8 cm × 10 cm collection of fluid behind the bladder containing a few bright echoes. Neither ovary was seen. What is the likely diagnosis?

11.5 What is the usual outcome?

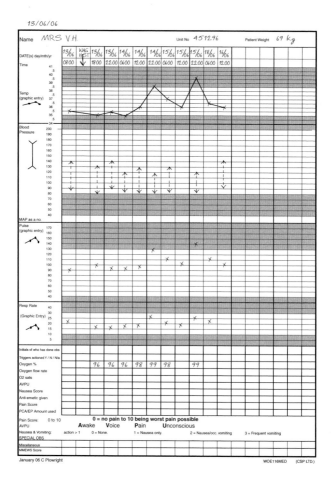

Mrs VP is a 63-year-old widow. She has been menopausal since the age of 50 and has not been sexually active since the death of her husband 8 years ago. She presents with a 6-month history of itching in vulval area. A photograph of her vulva is shown.

12.1 Describe the appearances of the vulva. Name two features.

12.2 What is the likely diagnosis?

12.3 How would you confirm your clinical diagnosis?

12.4 What is the first line of treatment? Name two preparations.

12.5 What other local treatment may improve symptoms? Name two.

12.6 List two radical treatments which may be used to treat severe intractable vulval pruritus.

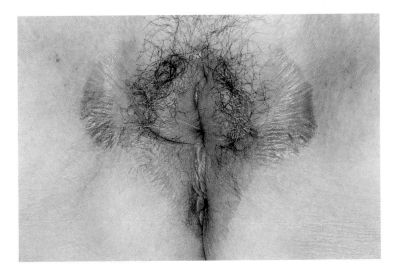

This 35-year-old woman presented with a 10-day history of pain and swelling in the right side of the vulva. The pain is throbbing and walking has become increasingly difficult. She also has an offensive vaginal discharge.

13.1 Which structure is involved?

13.2 What is the usual function of this structure?

13.3 What is the diagnosis?

13.4 How does this occur? State two mechanisms.

13.5 What are the principles of treatment? Name two.

13.6 What is this process called?

13.7 A swab from the pus drained shows Gram-negative intracellular diplococci. Where should the patient be referred?

13.8 Who else should be investigated?

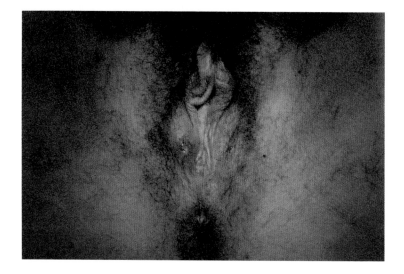

14.1 Define urinary incontinence. Specify two features.

14.2 A subtraction cystometric trace is shown. Name the abnormality which is demonstrated.

14.3 How may a woman with this result present? Specify two symptoms.

14.4 What simple measures may improve symptoms? Specify two.

14.5 Name two classes of drugs that may be of benefit.

14.6 Give an example of each class of drug (generic name with usual dose).

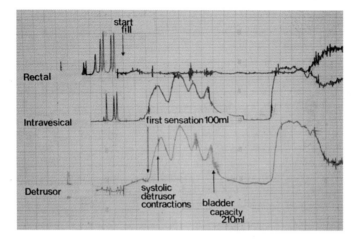

The photograph shows some commonly used preparations.

15.1 What is the generic term given to this group of preparations?

15.2 List two absolute contraindications to this treatment.

15.3 What are the long-term unseen benefits of such treatment? Name two.

15.4 What is the recommended minimum duration of therapy if long-term benefits are to be achieved?

15.5 In the non-hysterectomised woman, what are the alternatives to oral progestogen? Name two routes of administration.

15.6 What is meant by tachyphylaxis?

15.7 When using implants, how might you reduce tachyphylaxis?

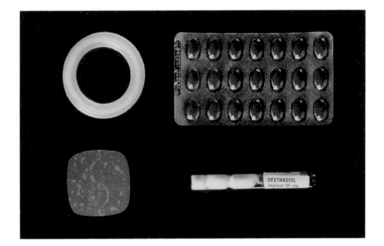

A gestational diabetic woman at term with a known large baby has been in the second stage of labour for 2 hours and you have been called to the room as she is delivering. When you walk into the room, the midwife says that she is unable to deliver all of the head. You look at the perineum and see a very blue face and make an instant diagnosis.

16.1 What is the diagnosis?

16.2 Mechanically, what has occurred?

16.3 How would you try to aid delivery?

16.4 In what percentage of cases should the manoeuvres described result in delivery?

16.5 Name and describe an internal rotatory manoeuvre.

16.6 Describe an alternative position for delivery.

16.7 All attempts to deliver have failed. Describe an option of last resort.

Mrs RM is in her third pregnancy. At her 38-week antenatal check by her midwife, she reports reduced fetal movements and her midwife advises her to fill in a kick chart.

17.1 What does the kick chart show?

17.2 List five causes of reduced fetal movements.

17.3 What non-invasive tests could you arrange for this woman to assess the well-being of her baby? List four tests.

- 13 -

FETAL MOVEMENT CHART   All Saints' Hospital
Tel: 01634 407311

Name ..... MRS R.M.

Address ....

Telephone ....

THE REASON FOR THIS CHART: This chart is to help us assess the health of your baby by finding out how active it is. At least 10 movements should be felt each day.

INSTRUCTIONS:
1. Start at 9.00am
2. When a movement is felt, make a tick in the box under 1st, 2nd, 3rd, etc. Several movements together should be classed as one.
3. Write down the time of the 10th movement.
4. If 10 movements are not felt by 6 pm ring All Saints' Hospital and ask to speak to the Liaison Midwife. She will make arrangements to monitor your baby.

START 9:00 AM

MOVEMENT OR KICKS

Date:	1st	2nd	3rd	4th	5th	6th	7th	8th	9th	10th+
Fri										
Sat										
Sun										
Mon										
11/9 Tue	✓	✓	✓	✓	✓	✓	✓	✓	✓	1.30 pm
12/9 Wed	✓	✓	✓	✓	✓	✓	✓	✓	✓	12.30 pm
13/9 Thu	✓	✓	✓	✓	✓	✓	✓	✓	✓	1.00 pm
14/9 Fri	✓	✓	✓	✓	✓	✓	✓	✓	✓	3.30 pm
15/9 Sat	✓	✓	✓	✓	✓	✓9.00 pm				
Sun										
Mon										
Tue										
Wed										
Thu										

OUCH!

GOAL!

A partogram is shown of a woman in her first labour.

18.1 When should charting of observations on a partogram be commenced?

18.2 What two criteria must be satisfied to make this diagnosis?

18.3 What abnormality is illustrated in the first stage of labour?

18.4 What intervention has been applied at A?

18.5 What has happened as a result of this intervention? State two consequences.

18.6 What is the minimum acceptable rate of cervical dilatation in the active phase of labour in a primiparous woman?

18.7 What other abnormality is illustrated?

18.8 How was this managed?

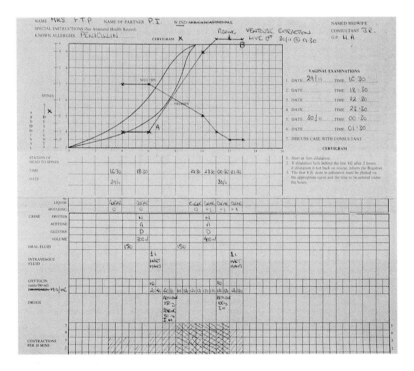

Look at the figure.
Please fill in the words that are missing, 1–10.

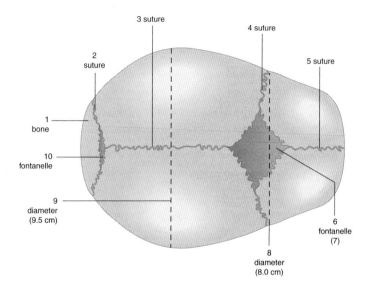

3 suture

4 suture

2 suture

5 suture

1 bone

10 fontanelle

9 diameter (9.5 cm)

6 fontanelle (7)

8 diameter (8.0 cm)

Mrs GD is 32 years old and in her fourth pregnancy. In her first pregnancy 14 years ago, she had an unexplained intrauterine death at 36 weeks. She has subsequently had two sons, aged 12 and 6, both by spontaneous vaginal delivery, weighing 4.2 and 4.6 kg at birth, respectively. At the 24- and 26-week antenatal visits, she had 2+ of glucose on urine analysis. Mrs GD's mother had maturity onset non-insulin-dependent diabetes. A 28-week, 75-g oral glucose tolerance test result is shown.

20.1 What is the diagnosis?

20.2 List four indications for a glucose tolerance test in Mrs GD's history.

20.3 Which blood test would reflect long-term glycaemia in this woman?

20.4 Name three other personnel whom you would involve in Mrs GD's management.

20.5 How would you control Mrs GD's glycaemia in labour?

Guy's Hospital **Department of Biochemistry**	Surname	D
	Forename	G
Date 11.10.06	Sex	F
	DOB	29.11.73
	Number	641129

Time	Blood Glucose
Fasting	4.9 mmol/l
60 minutes	11.3 mmol/l
120 minutes	15.1 mmol/l

1.1 Pyrexia 38.5°C, tachycardia 100–120/min, heavy vaginal loss/lochia [Marks 3]

1.2 Retained products of conception, endometritis [Marks 2]

1.3 Midstream urine for culture and sensitivity, blood culture, white cell count, endocervical swab/high vaginal swab [Marks 3]

1.4 Broad spectrum antibiotics [Marks 1]

1.5 Evacuation of retained products of conception [Marks 1]

2.1 There are two intrauterine gestation sacs, each containing a fetal pole [Marks 2]

2.2 Dichorionic, diamniotic [Marks 2]

2.3 Threatened miscarriage/threatened abortion [Marks 1]

2.4 Increased plasma volume, decreased red cell concentration, increased haematinic demand [Marks 2]

2.5 Increased maternal age, positive family history, ovulation induction/assisted conception [Marks 2]

2.6 No [Marks 1]

3.1 The anterior fontanelle/bregma [Marks 1]

3.2 Frontal and parietal bones [Marks 2]

3.3 Neonatal dehydration [Marks 1]

3.4 Increased intracranial tension/hydrocephalus/meningitis [Marks 1]

3.5 6 months [Marks 1]

3.6 Cephalhaematoma [Marks 1]

3.7 Haematoma that does not cross the suture lines [Marks 1]

3.8 Neonatal shock/anaemia, neonatal jaundice [Marks 2]

4.1   Mirena – progestogen-containing IUCD, Nova T [Marks 2]

4.2   Preventing implantation, promoting hostile cervical mucus, impeding sperm transport [Marks 2]

4.3   5 years, 5 years [Marks 2]

4.4   Pelvic infection, expulsion, perforation [Marks 2]

4.5   Copper allergy (Wilson's disease), PID, past history of tubal ectopic pregnancy in nulliparous women, distorted uterine activity [Marks 2]

5.1   Gram-negative diplococci [Marks 1]

5.2   Gonorrhoea [Marks 1]

5.3   Vaginal discharge, dysuria [Marks 2]

5.4   Mucopurulent cervical discharge [Marks 1]

5.5   Endocervix, urethra, rectum, pharynx [Marks 3]

5.6   Aqueous procaine penicillin 2.4–4.8 mu i.m. with or without probenecid 1 g orally, spectinomycin 2–4 g i.m., ampicillin 3 g orally with probenecid 1 g, cefadroxil 1 g by mouth, ciprofloxacin 500 g, doxycycline 300 mg by mouth, minocycline 300 mg by mouth [Marks 2]

6.1   The number of stillbirths and early neonatal deaths per 1000 livebirths and stillbirths [Marks 1]

6.2   5.7 per 1000 total births [Marks 1]

6.3   Congenital abnormality, antepartum haemorrhage, intrapartum causes [Marks 3]

6.4   30–34 years [Marks 1]

6.5   England, Wales and Northern Ireland [Marks 3]

6.6 1000 g [Marks 1]

6.7 Deaths occurring in labour or within up to 6 completed days of life [Marks 2]

Station 7	ANSWERS	Circuit B

7.1 Nausea, vomiting, epigastric pain, visual symptoms, headache [Marks 2]

7.2 Hyperreflexia, clonus, hepatic tenderness, optic fundi changes, hand and facial oedema [Marks 3]

7.3 High serum urate [Marks 1]

7.4 In hospital [Marks 1]

7.5 Cardiotocograph (CTG), USS, Doppler studies, biophysical profile [Marks 2]

7.6 Very low, <5% [Marks 1]

Station 8	ANSWERS	Circuit B

8.1 Placental abruption [Marks 1]

8.2 Clotting studies, U+E urate, urine for protein, CTG [Marks 3]

8.3 'Woody' hard/tense [Marks 1]

8.4 IV line/IV fluids, blood for cross match, urinary catheter, resuscitation if needed [Marks 3]

8.5 Institute delivery [Marks 1]

8.6 DIC [Marks 1]

Station 9	ANSWERS	Circuit B

9.1 Hirsutism [Marks1]

9.2 PCOS [Marks 1]

9.3 Luteinising hormone (LH), testosterone, oestrogen, androstenedione, dihydroepiandosterone (DHEA) [Marks 2]

9.4 Sex hormone binding globulin (SHBG) [Marks 1]

9.5 Ethinyl oestradiol and cyproterone acetate, dianette/low androgenic OC pill, advise weight reduction [Marks 2]

9.6 Endometrial pathology, cardiovascular disease, diabetes mellitus [Marks 1]

9.7 Thick smooth pearly white capsule, multiple small peripherally placed follicles, thecal cell hyperplasia [Marks 2]

Station 10   ANSWERS   Circuit B

10.1 Postcoital bleeding, intermenstrual bleeding [Marks 2]

10.2 Refer immediately for colposcopy, refer to gynaecologist for biopsy [Marks 1]

10.3 Wertheim's hysterectomy or radiotherapy [Marks 1]

10.4 Large number of sexual partners, HPV 16 and 18, smoking, previous cervical intraepithelial neoplasia (CIN), history of sexually transmitted disease (STD), early age of first coitus [Marks 4]

10.5 80% [Marks 1]

10.6 50–60 years [Marks 1]

Station 11   ANSWERS   Circuit B

11.1 Swinging pyrexia, tachycardia with pyrexia [Marks 2]

11.2 Examine the respiratory system/exclude pneumonia or atelectasis.
Examine the legs/exclude deep venous thrombosis.
Examine the wound/exclude wound infection, wound abscess.
Examine the vaginal vault/exclude vault haematoma.
Ballot kidneys/exclude pyelonephritis. [Marks 4]

11.3 Midstream urine for culture and sensitivity, wound swab for microscopy, culture and sensitivity, blood for culture and sensitivity, high vaginal swab for microscopy culture and sensitivity [Marks 2]

11.4 Infected vault haematoma [Marks 1]

11.5 Spontaneous drainage/resolution [Marks 1]

12.1 Papery thin atropic areas interspersed with reddened thick areas [Marks 2]

12.2 Lichen sclerosis et atrophicus [Marks 1]

12.3 Skin biopsy and histological analysis/examination [Marks 1]

12.4 Topical glucocorticoids/hydrocortisone, dermovate/betnovate/betamethasone [Marks 2]

12.5 Topical oestrogen cream/local anaesthetic/topical 2% testosterone [Marks 2]

12.6 Radiotherapy, skinning vulvectomy/simple vulvectomy [Marks 2]

13.1 Bartholin's gland [Marks 1]

13.2 Secretion of mucoid fluid for lubrication [Marks 1]

13.3 Bartholin's abscess [Marks 1]

13.4 Duct of Bartholin's gland becomes blocked, mucoid secretion collects and becomes infected [Marks 2]

13.5 Deroofing the Bartholin's abscess to drain off pus, maintaining duct patency to encourage ongoing drainage [Marks 2]

13.6 Marsupialisation [Marks 1]

13.7 Genitourinary medicine clinic/STD clinic [Marks 1]

13.8 The woman's partner(s) [Marks 1]

14.1 This is a condition in which there is involuntary loss of urine, leading to a social or personal problem with hygiene [Marks 1]

14.2 Detrusor instability [Marks 1]

14.3 Stress incontinence/urge incontinence, frequency/urgency/dysuria, nocturia/enuresis [Marks 2]

14.4 Bladder drill/bladder training, reduction in fluid intake, especially in the evening, avoidance of caffeine [Marks 2]

14.5 Anticholinergic drugs, antimuscarinics [Marks 2]

14.6 Propantheline hydrochloride 15 mg b.d., oxybutynin 2.5 mg b.d., imipramine 25 mg b.d. – anticholinergics; tolterodine 4 mg daily, solifenacin 5 mg daily – antimuscarinics [Marks 2]

Station 15	ANSWERS	Circuit B

15.1 Hormone replacement therapy [Marks 1]

15.2 Oestrogen-dependent tumour/breast carcinoma/endometrial carcinoma, active liver disease/chronic active hepatitis/acute hepatitis, undiagnosed abnormal vaginal bleeding [Marks 2]

15.3 Prevention of osteoporosis/bone loss/preservation of bone, prevention of colorectal cancer [Marks 2]

15.4 At least 5 years [Marks 1]

15.5 Transdermal progestogen, intrauterine progesterone-containing device, vaginal progestogen [Marks 2]

15.6 Return of symptoms despite high levels of drug/oestrogen [Marks 1]

15.7 Measure serum oestradiol prior to administration, strict adherence to time of giving implants (i.e. not less than 6 months apart) [Marks 1]

Station 16	ANSWERS	Circuit B

16.1 Shoulder dystocia [Marks 1]

16.2 The anterior shoulder has impacted above the symphysis pubis or, less commonly, the posterior shoulder has impacted above the sacral promontory [Marks 2]

16.3 Episiotomy, McRobert's manoeuvre, deliver posterior arm, suprapubic pressure [Marks 2]

16.4 80%–90% [Marks 1]

16.5 Rubin's manoeuvre: fingers behind anterior shoulder rotate towards fetal chest. Fingers of other hand press in front of posterior shoulder = Wood's screw. Also reverse Wood's screw [Marks 2]

16.6 All fours position or left lateral position [Marks 1]

16.7 Symphisiotomy, Zavanelli manoeuvre (cephalic replacement) and fetal clavicular fracture [Marks 1]

Station 17	ANSWERS	Circuit B

17.1 Reduced fetal movements: six movements in 12 hours [Marks 1]

17.2 Normal sleep phase, physiological (towards the end of pregnancy), reduced maternal perception (idiopathic or due to distraction), sedative drugs given to mother (e.g. barbiturates), polyhydramnios/oligohydramnios, intrauterine asphyxia [Marks 5]

17.3 Cardiotocography (non-stress), ultrasound for fetal growth and liquor, formal biophysical profile, umbilical artery Doppler studies/velocimetry [Marks 4]

Station 18	ANSWERS	Circuit B

18.1 When labour is established/has reached the active phase, when diagnosis of labour has been made [Marks 1]

18.2 Regular uterine contractions accompanied by progressive cervical change [Marks 2]

18.3 Primary uterine inertia/prolonged first stage/delayed progress in first stage/primary arrest [Marks 1]

18.4 Oxytocin infusion [Marks 1]

18.5 Increase in intensity/frequency/duration of contractions, acceleration of cervical dilatation [Marks 2]

18.6 More than or equal to 1 cm/hour [Marks 1]

18.7 Secondary arrest/prolonged second stage [Marks 1]

18.8 Ventouse extraction/operative vaginal delivery [Marks 1]

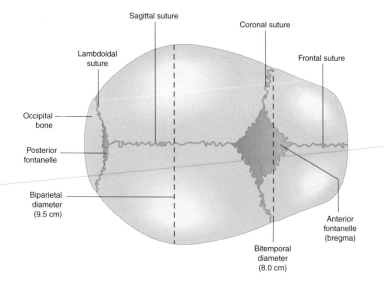

20.1 Diabetes mellitus in pregnancy [Marks 1]

20.2 Family history of diabetes mellitus, unexplained IUD, previous fetal macrosomia, persistent glycosuria [Marks 4]

20.3 Glycosolated haemoglobin/haemoglobin A1C/fructosamine [Marks 1]

20.4 Consultant endocrinologist/diabetologist, diabetic specialist nurse/midwife, dietician [Marks 3]

20.5 Continuous glucose infusion together with sliding scale insulin infusion [Marks 1]

Objective structured clinical examination (OSCEs)

Circuit C

1.1 Name four advantages of the method of contraception shown below.

1.2 Name four disadvantages.

1.3 If this method failed during intercourse, what would you advise for emergency contraception? Name constituent(s) and dose.

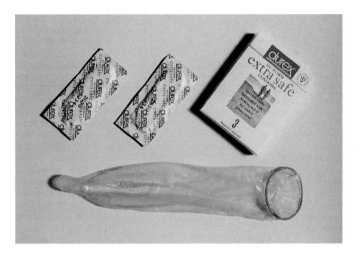

Mrs AM is 39 weeks pregnant in her third pregnancy.
Her antenatal hepatitis B screening result is shown.

2.1   Specify four mechanisms by which hepatitis B infection may be
          transmitted.

2.2   What grade of infectivity does the blood result imply?

2.3   What three measures would you recommend for this woman's
          newborn baby?

2.4   How soon should the newborn baby be immunised?

2.5   Of those babies infected perinatally, what percentage will become
          chronic carriers?

Guy's Hospital **Department of Virology**	Surname	M
	Forename	A
Date 19.7.06	Sex	F
	DOB	2.2.68
	Number	S80202

Hepatitis B surface antigen detected
e antigen detected
e antibody negative

The table shows deaths from hypertensive disorders of pregnancy in the UK between 1985 and 2002.

3.1   Comment on the two trends shown.

3.2   In 2000–2002, substandard care was identified in 50% of cases. How does this compare with previous triennia?

3.3   Two factors have consistently been identified as contributing to the substandard care. What are these?

3.4   What is now considered to be the anticonvulsant of choice in eclampsia and pre-eclampsia?

3.5   What was the commonest cause of death from pre-eclampsia/ eclampsia?

3.6   In the latest maternal mortality report (2000–2002), where did hypertensive diseases rate among the commonest causes of direct deaths?

3.7   List three practice points which are recommended to reduce the risks of pulmonary complications.

The number of women who died from hypertensive disorders of pregnancy in the 6 triennia from 1985 to 2002		
Triennium	Number of deaths	Death rate (per million pregnancies)
1985–1987	27	11.9
1988–1990	27	11.4
1991–1993	20	8.6
1994–1996	20	9.1
1997–1999	15	7.1
2000–2002	14	7.0
Adapted from CEMACH 2000–2002, Department of Health		

Mrs EF has been attending your GP surgery for her antenatal care and her antenatal records are shown.

4.1 With regards to BP in pregnancy, what normally happens in the first trimester?

4.2 What happens in the second trimester normally?

4.3 What happens in the third trimester normally?

4.4 What features are you concerned about with Mrs EF? Name two.

4.5 What do you arrange now? Name five measures.

Mrs EF LMP 6/12/05		Antenatal Record EDD 12/09/06								DOB 10/1/74	
Date	Gestation	Problems	SFH	Position	Descent of head	Fetal heart	BP	Urine Prot.	CIU.	Comment	Seen by & date
27/2/06	11	–	–	–	–	–	$\frac{110}{70}$	–	–	Delighted	2/4
2/4/06	16	Nil	–	–	–	–	$\frac{100}{60}$	–	–	Tired	25/4
25/4/06	20	Nil	20 cm	–	–	Heard	$\frac{110}{60}$	–	–	Feels fine	22/5
22/5/06	24	Nil	24 cm	–	–	Heard	$\frac{120}{70}$	–	–	All well	21/6
21/6/06	28	Nil	27 cm	Ceph.	5/5	Heard	$\frac{120}{70}$	–	–	Fine	19/7
19/7/06	32	Tired	31 cm	Ceph.	4/5	Heard	$\frac{150}{95}$	1+	–		

You are called to the labour ward 15 minutes after a para 3 gravida 4 has had a normal delivery. She is bleeding excessively.

5.1 What is the first thing you do when you enter the room (apart from introducing yourself)?

5.2 What two relevant questions do you ask the midwife?

5.3 What do you then do? Name five courses of action.

5.4 What is the most likely cause?

5.5 You are unable to stop the bleeding. What measure do you take while awaiting senior help?

Part of Ms HP's antenatal care chart is shown.

6.1   List five features that place her in a high-risk category for
pregnancy which would have been identified at the booking visit.

6.2   Comment on her 24 and 26 weeks visits to her midwife.

6.3   What investigation would you have arranged?

6.4   She is seen in the hospital antenatal clinic around 32/40.
Comment on the abdominal findings.

6.5   What investigation would you arrange at this visit?

6.6   At 38/40, Ms HP is delivered of a 2.1-kg baby boy by LSCS.
Comment on this.

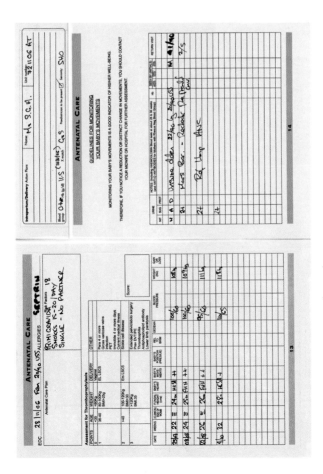

Mrs PB had a Neville–Barnes forceps delivery for a prolonged second stage in her first pregnancy 6 days ago. She has been suffering with perineal pain since the delivery, which has not improved, and it continues to be painful to sit or open her bowels. A photograph of her perineum is shown.

7.1 What has happened?

7.2 List four factors which may predispose to this complication.

7.3 In the absence of infection, how is this complication best managed? Specify two points.

7.4 List three simple measures which may improve symptoms.

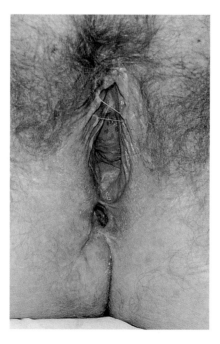

A 19-year-old girl presents with primary amenorrhoea. She has a webbed neck and a wide carrying angle. She is 141 cm. An X-ray of her hands is shown.

8.1 What abnormality is shown?

8.2 What is the most likely diagnosis?

8.3 If you analysed her chromosomes, what would they show?

8.4 What hormone test would you request?

8.5 What would her uterus look like?

8.6 What would her gonads look like?

8.7 What hormonal replacement would you give her?

8.8 Name two conditions under which this woman could become pregnant.

8.9 Name one way this condition could have been detected during her mother's pregnancy.

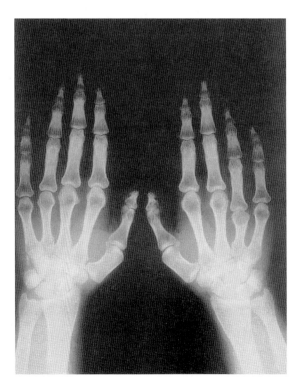

This 76-year-old woman presented with soreness of the vulva.

9.1 What do you see?

9.2 What is the most likely diagnosis?

9.3 What is the most common histological diagnosis?

9.4 Which nodes would this spread to?

9.5 What is the treatment of choice? Name two components.

9.6 What is the 5-year survival rate for node negative stage 1 cases?

9.7 Name three predisposing factors for this condition.

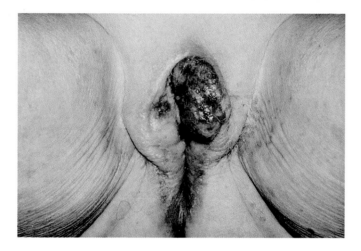

This photograph was taken laparoscopically.

10.1 What abnormality does it show?

10.2 Name three symptoms this patient may have presented with.

10.3 If she was to have this abnormality removed by a conservative procedure, what intraoperative complications may arise? Name two.

10.4 What must a patient be warned about prior to this operation?

10.5 If this woman had become pregnant prior to her operation, name two complications that she may have had during the pregnancy.

10.6 In what percentage of cases may this condition be malignant?

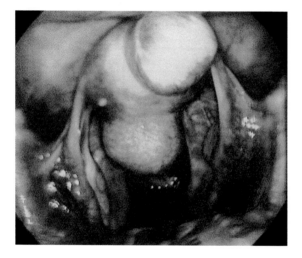

Mrs CD is a 35-year-old housewife with two children. She was sterilised 2 years ago and since the operation her periods have been very heavy. Her GP performed a cervical smear and the result is shown.

11.1 What does the result suggest?

11.2 What investigation is indicated? Name two features.

11.3 Name two solutions used to identify abnormal areas on the cervix.

11.4 The squamo-columnar junction is wholly visible and biopsy of a clearly defined abnormal area confirms CIN II. List three methods suitable for removing the abnormal area.

11.5 If the extent of the abnormal area is not visible, which diagnostic procedure is indicated?

11.6 Given Mrs CD's menstrual history, what other surgical options should be considered? Name one.

An X-ray is shown.

12.1 What is this investigation called?

12.2 Describe the findings. Specify two features.

12.3 What is the commonest microorganism leading to this picture?

12.4 In the presence of normal ovulation and a normal semen analysis in her partner, what are the two options for facilitating conception in this patient?

12.5 What is the usually quoted take-home baby rate following in vitro fertilisation in experienced hands?

12.6 List three important complications of IVF.

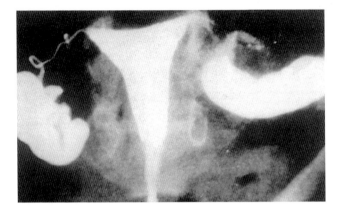

A 22-year-old woman who has recently married complained of deep dyspareunia on every occasion of coitus. She also reports a copious inoffensive discharge and occasional postcoital bleeding. She uses the combined oral contraceptive pill and has regular withdrawal bleeds.

13.1   List three investigations you would arrange during your speculum examination.

13.2   Speculum examination reveals a florid ectropion. Which of her symptoms might this cause? Name two.

13.3   If the investigations performed in Question 13.1 were normal, how would you treat the ectropion?

13.4   Name the structure shown below.

13.5   What is this used for?

13.6   Use of this structure results in the alleviation of symptoms. Which operation would you recommend?

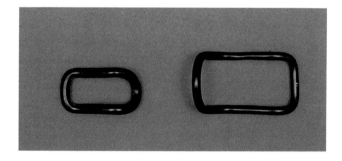

14.1 Look at the result shown. Name the investigation.

14.2 Define a normal urinary flow rate for a woman.

14.3 What is the abnormality shown?

14.4 What simple measures may improve the patient's symptoms? Name two.

14.5 List three surgical approaches to treat this condition, and provide an example of each.

14.6 Which operation has the highest documented success rate?

14.7 What is the usually quoted success rate in experienced hands?

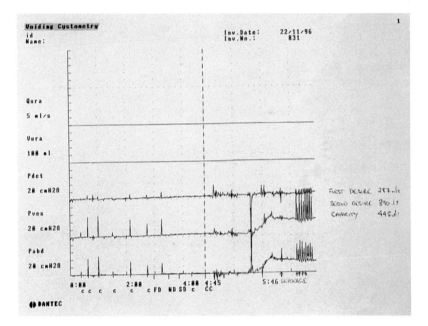

A 34-year-old lady presents to her GP at 27 weeks in her first pregnancy complaining of lower abdominal pain.

15.1 Give three possible uterine causes of the pain.

15.2 Give three possible non-uterine causes of the pain.

15.3 What clinical signs would you look for on examination to help you make a diagnosis? Name four.

This station concerns drugs in pregnancy.

16.1 Define the term teratogen.

16.2 What is the approximate molecular weight of substances which readily cross the placenta?

16.3 List the three phases of development of a conceptus and specify the precise timing in completed weeks post-conception.

16.4 At which of these phases does exposure to a teratogen have the greatest potential to cause gross malformation?

16.5 What criteria must be satisfied before prescribing a pregnant woman a known teratogen?

17.1   What is the incidence of spontaneous twins in the UK?

17.2   This incidence is rising. Why?

17.3   What percentage of spontaneous twins are monozygotic?

17.4   Graphs 1 and 2 (A) show serial ultrasound measurements of abdominal and head circumference in a monochorionic–diamniotic twin pregnancy. Describe three findings.

17.5   Graph 3 (B) shows serial amniotic fluid index measurements from the two sacs. Describe two findings.

17.6   What term is used to describe this sequence of events?

17.7   Umbilical arterial Doppler of twin 2 shows reversed end diastolic flow. What would you arrange?

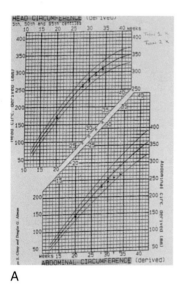

A

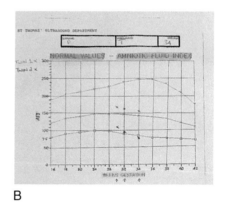

B

Miss PL is a 15-year-old school girl who is 29 weeks pregnant. She has previously had an evacuation termination of pregnancy at 15 weeks gestation for social reasons. She has smoked since the age of 11 and lives with her unemployed divorced mother on income support. She presents to the labour ward with a 3-hour history of painful contractions every 10 minutes.

18.1 Define preterm delivery.

18.2 What is the incidence of preterm delivery?

18.3 List four risk factors for preterm delivery in Miss PL's history.

18.4 What examinations would you carry out to establish a diagnosis of preterm labour? Specify two.

18.5 In the presence of preterm labour, what would you administer to Miss PL to encourage fetal lung maturation? Specify preparation, dose, route of administration and frequency.

A 26-year-old woman presents to the antenatal clinic at 18 weeks gestation and the subject of HIV antenatal testing is discussed with her. She agrees to have the test as her previous partner was bisexual. The results come back positive and termination is discussed. She declines termination.

19.1 What would you advise her about the rate of vertical transmission?

19.2 During the pregnancy, her CD4 count is <200 mm³ on three occasions. What would you give her for prophylaxis against *Pneumocystis carinii* pneumonia (PCP)?

19.3 Women diagnosed as HIV positive during pregnancy should be managed by a multidisciplinary team. Ideally who should be in this team? Name four.

19.4 State three interventions to reduce the risk of vertical transmission from mother to baby.

19.5 If the above three interventions are implemented, what is the associated vertical transmission rate?

19.6 How long does it take for the baby to lose maternal antibody?

19.7 What immunisations should the baby not be given? Name two.

Miss EP was referred to A&E with a 6.5-week history of amenorrhoea and left iliac fossa pain. A urinary BHCG was positive and a transvaginal ultrasound scan was performed, shown below.

20.1 Describe the appearance of the uterine cavity.

20.2 Describe the finding to the left of the uterus.

20.3 Where is the answer to Question 20.2 likely to be located?

20.4 Miss EP is haemodynamically stable with no signs of peritonism. State four different methods of treating her condition.

20.5 If a laparoscopic conservative procedure is performed, when would you expect Miss EP to be well enough to go home?

20.6 How should she be followed up?

20.7 What is currently the most common aetiological factor associated with ectopic pregnancy?

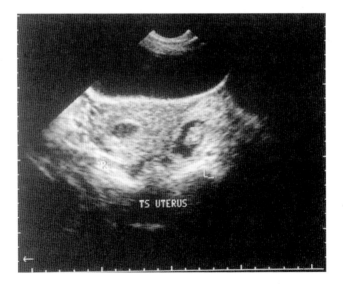

TS UTERUS

1.1 Protection against STD, protection from carcinoma of the cervix, no systemic side-effects, easily available, instantly effective [Marks 4]

1.2 Requires continuous motivation, action required at time of coitus, user failure can be high, decreased sensation in the male, latex allergies [Marks 4]

1.3 Levonelle 750 mg. Levonorgestrel within 72 hours of unprotected sexual intercourse and another dose 12 hours later. Insert an IUCD within 5 days of intercourse [Marks 2]

2.1 Sexually/anal intercourse/vaginal intercourse, parenterally/blood transfusion/needle stick, perinatal transmission/vertical transmission, breastfeeding, blood splash on open wound/eyes [Marks 4]

2.2 High infectivity [Marks 1]

2.3 Active immunisation/hepatitis B vaccination, passive immunisation/hepatitis B immunoglobin, avoidance of breastfeeding if possible [Marks 3]

2.4 Within 24 hours [Marks 1]

2.5 90% [Marks 1]

3.1 There is a fall in both absolute numbers of deaths and the rates of death per million maternities over the triennia [Marks 2]

3.2 Improvement [Marks 1]

3.3 Failure to take prompt action, inadequate/late consultant involvement [Marks 2]

3.4 Magnesium sulphate [Marks 1]

3.5 Cerebral (intracranial) haemorrhage [Marks 1]

3.6 Third [Marks 1]

3.7 Accurate fluid balance measurement, fluid restriction and central venous pressure monitoring [Marks 2]

4.1 BP drops [Marks 1]

4.2 BP drops more significantly [Marks 1]

4.3 BP returns to first trimester levels [Marks 1]

4.4 BP has risen significantly at 32 weeks, proteinuria has developed [Marks 2]

4.5 MSU, FBC, serum urate, refer to day assessment unit 24-hour urinary protein estimation [Marks 5]

5.1 Rub up a contraction [Marks 1]

5.2 Has she had ergometrine or Syntocinon with the anterior shoulder? Was the placenta complete? [Marks 2]

5.3 Call senior help, i.v. line, blood for cross match, FBC, Syntocinon/ergometrine, clotting studies [Marks 5]

5.4 Atonic uterus [Marks 1]

5.5 Bimanual compression [Marks 1]

6.1 Primigravida, smoker, maternal weight >100 g, unsupported/ (single mother), unsure dates, 18 years of age [Marks 5]

6.2 Persistent 2 + glycosuria [Marks 1]

6.3 Oral glucose tolerance test (GTT) [Marks 1]

6.4 Clinically small for dates [Marks 1]

6.5 USS for growth and liquor [Marks 1]

6.6 Confirmed small for gestational age baby [Marks 1]

7.1 Partial breakdown of episiotomy repair [Marks 1]

7.2 Poor repair technique, perineal wound haematoma, perineal wound infection, poor hygiene after repair, undiagnosed third degree tear, maternal diabetes, HIV infection [Marks 4]

7.3 Careful hygiene/surgical toilet, allow healing by secondary intention/granulation [Marks 2]

7.4 Simple analgesia, anti-inflammatory drugs, stool softeners, inflatable rubber ring (to sit on) [Marks 3]

8.1 Shortened 4th metacarpal of the left hand [Marks 1]

8.2 Turner's syndrome [Marks 1]

8.3 XO [Marks 1]

8.4 Follicle stimulating hormone (FSH) [Marks 1]

8.5 Rudimentary/hypoplastic [Marks 1]

8.6 Absent or streak ovaries [Marks 1]

8.7 Oestrogen and progestogens/COC pill/HRT [Marks 1]

8.8 If she was a Turner's mosaic, oocyte donation [Marks 2]

8.9 USS, amniocentesis, chorionic villous sampling (CVS) [Marks 1]

9.1 Tumour on the vulva [Marks 1]

9.2 Vulva carcinoma [Marks 1]

9.3 Squamous carcinoma [Marks 1]

9.4 Inguinal and femoral nodes, deep pelvic nodes [Marks 1]

9.5 Radical vulvectomy and bilateral groin node dissection [Marks 2]

9.6 95% [Marks 1]

9.7 Chronic vulval irritation, premalignant disease of vagina, premalignant disease of cervix [Marks 3]

Station 10	ANSWERS	Circuit C

10.1 Fibroid uterus [Marks 1]

10.2 Abdominal distension, infertility, difficulty with micturition, abdominal pain, menorrhagia [Marks 3]

10.3 Haemorrhage, damage to other organs, e.g. ureter, bladder, bowel [Marks 2]

10.4 A blood transfusion and/or hysterectomy may be needed [Marks 1]

10.5 Abnormal lie, urinary retention, placental abruption/APH [Marks 2]

10.6 0.2% [Marks 1]

Station 11	ANSWERS	Circuit C

11.1 Premalignant disease of the cervix/cervical precancer [Marks 1]

11.2 Colposcopy, colposcopic biopsy [Marks 2]

11.3 Acetic acid, Lugol's iodine/iodine [Marks 2]

11.4 Cold coagulation, diathermy ablation, diathermy excision, laser ablation, LLETZ [Marks 3]

11.5 Knife cone biopsy, large loop cone, laser cone biopsy [Marks 1]

11.6 Total abdominal hysterectomy, vaginal hysterectomy [Marks 1]

Station 12	ANSWERS	Circuit C

12.1 Hysterosalpingogram [Marks 1]

12.2 Normal outline of the uterine cavity, dilated tubal lumen; no spillage, bilateral hydrosalpinges [Marks 2]

12.3 Chlamydia (trachomatis) [Marks 1]

12.4 Tubal surgery/microsurgery/salpingostomy, in vitro fertilisation [Marks 2]

12.5 20–30% [Marks 1]

12.6 Ovarian hyperstimulation, multiple pregnancy, ectopic pregnancy, miscarriage, failed conception, congenital malformation [Marks 3]

Station 13 ANSWERS Circuit **C**

13.1 Cervical smear, endocervical swab for chlamydia, high vaginal swab for microscopy culture and sensitivity [Marks 3]

13.2 Discharge, postcoital bleeding, dyspareunia in the presence of cervicitis [Marks 2]

13.3 Cryocautery/cold coagulation/diathermy/laser [Marks 1]

13.4 Hodge pessary [Marks 1]

13.5 Reversible anteversion of a mobile retroverted uterus [Marks 2]

13.6 Ventrosuspension [Marks 1]

Station 14 ANSWERS Circuit **C**

14.1 Subtraction cystometry and uroflowmetry/urodynamic studies [Marks 1]

14.2 >15 ml/s [Marks 1]

14.3 Genuine stress incontinence [Marks 1]

14.4 Weight loss, stop smoking, treat constipation, pelvic floor exercises, physiotherapy, faradism, vaginal cones [Marks 2]

14.5 Vaginal approach, e.g. tension-free vaginal tape or transobturator tape; abdominal approach, e.g. Burch colposuspension/tension-free vaginal tape; combined abdominovaginal approach, e.g. suburethral fascial sling or Aldridge sling [Marks 3]

14.6 Colposuspension/TVT [Marks 1]

14.7 80–90% [Marks 1]

15.1 Preterm labour, abruption, fibroid degeneration, chorioamnionitis [Marks 3]

15.2 Urinary tract infection (UTI), constipation, appendicitis, ovarian cyst (accident), gastroenteritis, inflammatory bowel disease [Marks 3]

15.3 Pyrexia, tachycardia/hypotension/shock; uterus – soft or tense/ contractions/tender; vaginal examination – cervical change (effacing, dilatation)/evidence of SROM/discharge; abdominal – tenderness/guarding; renal angle tenderness [Marks 4]

16.1 A teratogen is a substance that causes structural or functional abnormality in a fetus exposed to that substance [Marks 1]

16.2 Molecular weight less than 1000 [Marks 1]

16.3 Pre-embryonic phase: 0–2 weeks, embryonic phase: 3–8 weeks, fetal phase: 9 weeks to birth [Marks 6]

16.4 Embryonic phase [Marks 1]

16.5 The potential benefit(s) to the mother must outweigh or justify the risk to the fetus [Marks 1]

17.1 1:80 [Marks 1]

17.2 As a result of assisted conception/ovulation induction regimens [Marks 1]

17.3 28–30% [Marks 1]

17.4 Twin 1 is growing normally along the 50th centile.
Twin 2 has a decreasing abdominal circumference.
Twin 2 has a normal head circumference (accept head sparing/ asymmetrical growth retardation). [Marks 3]

17.5 Twin 1 has normal liquor.
Twin 2 has reduced liquor/oligohydramnios. [Marks 2]

17.6 IUGR in twin 2 [Marks 1]

17.7 Emergency lower segment caesarean section.
Fetal cord blood sample. [Marks 1]

18.1 This is delivery occurring after 24 completed weeks of gestation but prior to 37 completed weeks of gestation [Marks 1]

18.2 Approximately 10% of all deliveries [Marks 1]

18.3 Age <16 years, cigarette smoking, low socioeconomic class, previous mid-trimester evacuation termination [Marks 4]

18.4 Abdominal palpation (to assess intensity frequency and duration of contractions), serial cervical assessment (to assess change in effacement/consistency/dilatation of the cervix) [Marks 2]

18.5 Dexamethasone 12 mg i.m. (two doses separated by 12 hours), or betamethasone 12 mg i.m. (two doses separated by 12 hours) [Marks 2]

19.1 15–20% in the non-breastfeeding population and breastfeeding doubles the risk [Marks 1]

19.2 Cotrimoxazole 960 mg daily on 3 days a week [Marks 1]

19.3 Obstetrician with a special interest in the disease, an HIV physician, an interested midwife, an interested neonatal paediatrician and a psychiatric team/patient support person [Marks 2]

19.4 Antiretroviral therapy given antenatally and intrapartum to the mother and to the neonate for the first 4–6 weeks of life; delivery by caesarean section avoidance of breastfeeding [Marks 3]

19.5 Less than 2% [Marks 1]

19.6 Up to 18 months [Marks 1]

19.7 Live oral polio vaccine, as there is a theoretical risk of causing persistent infection in children or harm to HIV-infected family members; BCG [Marks 1]

20.1 A central sac in the uterus (pseudosac) [Marks 1]

20.2 A true gestation sac with an identifiable fetus [Marks 1]

20.3 In the left fallopian tube [Marks 1]

20.4 Intravenous methothrexate, intratubal methothrexate guided by ultrasound, intratubal saline/methothrexate under laparoscopic control, laparoscopic salpingotomy/salpingectomy, laparotomy and salpingotomy/salpingectomy [Marks 4]

20.5 Within 24 hours/the next day [Marks 1]

20.6 With serial serum BHCG quantitation separated by 48–72 hours [Marks 1]

20.7 Pelvic inflammatory disease/chlamydia infection [Marks 1]

Objective structured clinical examination (OSCEs)

Circuit D

1.1 What eponym is given to this test?

1.2 Specify two features which would lead you to suspect an abnormal result.

1.3 Name the condition that this test is designed to detect.

1.4 How common is this condition?

1.5 What percentage of babies with an abnormal screening test result actually have the condition?

1.6 Is there a sex difference in incidence? Please specify.

1.7 Name an important obstetric risk factor.

1.8 If the screening test is positive, to whom should the baby be referred?

1.9 In the presence of a persistently abnormal result, what is the first line of treatment?

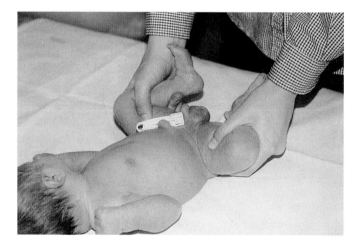

2.1   What object is seen?

2.2   What does this object do?

2.3   What other objects can be used? Name two.

2.4   What is this procedure called?

2.5   What is the failure rate of this procedure?

2.6   Name two points you would ensure the couple understood about the procedure.

2.7   Name two reasons for this procedure failing.

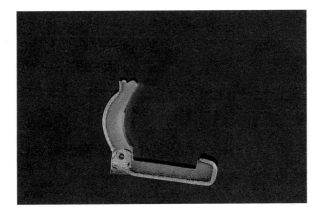

3.1 Describe what you see.

3.2 What is this syndrome called?

3.3 What is the most likely organism?

3.4 In the outpatients' department, what specimen would you take to detect this organism?

3.5 Name two antibiotics to which this organism is sensitive.

3.6 If a neonate is exposed to chlamydia, what may he/she develop?

3.7 If a male had this organism, name the clinical diagnosis.

3.8 What other organism may cause the above appearance?

3.9 What is the treatment?

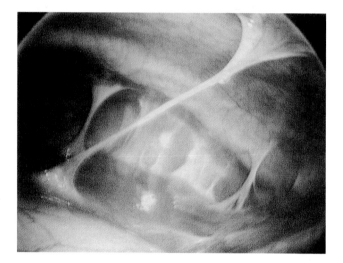

4.1   What do the letters NCEPOD stand for?

4.2   In which year did this enquiry commence?

4.3   What was the original title?

4.4   Which data were included in the early enquiries?

In 2003 a report entitled Who Operates When II (WOW II) was published. There was direct comparison to WOW I (1997). For the cohort studied a total of 9210 non-elective cases were analysed. A total of 921 of these were in gynaecology. The following table shows the time the procedures were carried out.

Time of surgery	Weekday 0800–1759	1800–2359	Weekend 0800–1759	1800–2359	Night 0000–0759
No of patients	533	207	96	31	41

4.5   What percentage of gynaecology non-elective cases were performed outside of normal working hours?

4.6   What percentage of gynaecology non-elective cases were performed at night?

The next table shows the grade of surgeon performing non-elective cases by the time of day. Values are given in percentages.

	Day WOW I	WOW II	Evening WOW I	WOW II	Night WOW I	WOW II
Consultant	28.5%	41.4%	14.2%	20.6%	11.4%	25.6%
SAS	7.3%	14.5%	5.9%	16.1%	5.6%	11.5%
SPR3+	13.3%	14.1%	13.1%	19.4%	15.0%	22.1%
SPR1–2	33.0%	11.0%	41.5%	13.9%	42.9%	13.5%
SHO	13.4%	5.0%	21.9%	9.0%	22.3%	6.6%
Other/blank	4.5%	14.0%	3.4%	21.0%	2.8%	20.6%

4.7   In WOW II what percentage of non-elective cases performed at night were performed by a junior trainee (SHO and SPR2)?

4.8   In WOW II what percentage of non-elective cases were performed by senior trainees (SPR3+), SAS and Consultants?

4.9   How does the figure for 4.8 compare with WOW I?

A sample of urine is provided from a 32-week primigravida patient with BP 160/100 mmHg, with no past history of note. The urine is tested with BM stix.

5.1 What substance has been detected?

5.2 What is the concentration in grams per litre?

5.3 What other maternal investigations would you arrange? Name five.

5.4 What is your management?

5.5 Name the two most likely diagnoses.

The specimen was produced from a postpartum hysterectomy. The woman had uterine inversion during the third stage.

6.1   What caused the uterine inversion? Name two problems.

6.2   How do you initially manage uterine inversion?

6.3   If your first manoeuvre fails, what do you do?

6.4   Why do you think this woman had a hysterectomy?

6.5   Name three intraoperative complications that may occur during a postpartum hysterectomy.

6.6   Would the ovaries be removed at the time of operation?

6.7   Name one predisposing factor to the underlying pathology.

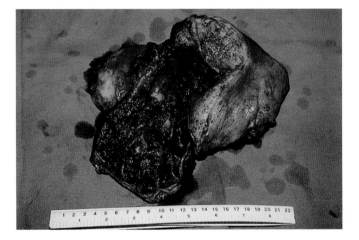

Mrs AS is a 22-year-old Nigerian woman in her first pregnancy. Her booking haemoglobin electrophoresis result is shown.

7.1   What haemoglobinopathy does Mrs AS have?

7.2   Who else should be tested?

7.3   If Mrs AS's partner also has the same haemoglobinopathy, what are the respective chances of the fetus being normal, having the same haemoglobinopathy as either parent or the overt disease?

7.4   What has been the usual method for prenatal diagnosis of haemoglobinopathy in the fetus? Specify the tissue sample and the test.

7.5   At what gestation is this usually performed?

7.6   State two other sources of DNA which allow earlier diagnosis of haemoglobinopathy.

Guy's Hospital **Department of Haematology**	Surname	S
	Forename	A
Date 27.10.06	Sex	F
	DOB	27.9.84
	Number	630927

Haemoglobin Electrophoresis

H6 A	65%
H6 S	30%
H6 F	3%

Mrs ST had a normal delivery of a baby boy 2 weeks ago. She has been breastfeeding her son and has recently developed 'flu-like' symptoms. Her left breast has become swollen and painful, and on examination she has a temperature of 38.2°C but there is no sign of an upper respiratory tract infection. A photograph of her breasts is shown.

8.1   Describe the appearance of the left breast.

8.2   What is the diagnosis?

8.3   What is the usual infective organism?

8.4   How is this best treated? Give the name of the preparation, and the route, dose and frequency.

8.5   Specify two factors which may contribute to this clinical picture.

8.6   Mrs ST develops a purulent exudate from her left nipple. What should you advise? Name two features.

8.7   What further complication is she at risk from?

8.8   If this latter complication occurs, how should it be treated?

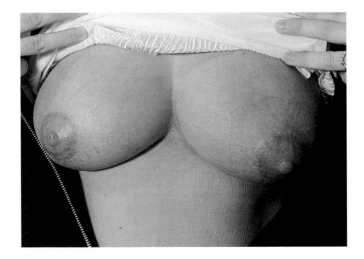

Mrs MA is a Caucasian woman in her second pregnancy. She has a 1-year-old girl and has not had a period for 13 weeks. She initially suffered with severe nausea but this subsequently resolved and she has been well for the last 4 weeks. During the past 48 hours, she has been experiencing a dark brown vaginal loss. A transvaginal ultrasound scan has been performed and a photograph of the findings is shown.

9.1 Describe the findings in the uterine cavity. Name two features.

9.2 What embryonic measurement is shown?

9.3 State the numerical value of the measurement and the corresponding gestational age.

9.4 During real-time scanning, the fetal heart is identified but is not seen beating. What is the diagnosis?

9.5 Which two haematological tests would you arrange?

9.6 Name the procedure that is indicated and the usual anaesthetic used.

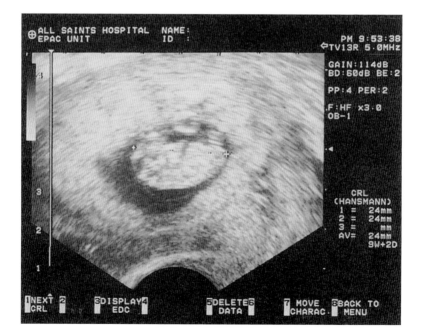

Mrs HF is 23 years old and in her second pregnancy. A blood result taken at 12 weeks by her midwife is shown.

10.1 What does the blood result show?

10.2 What proportion of the UK population have rhesus-negative blood?

10.3 In the presence of a rhesus-positive fetus, what condition may affect the fetus as a result of this level of anti-D antibody in the maternal serum?

10.4 Which immunoglobulin is responsible for the condition in the fetus?

10.5 What antigen does it bond to?

10.6 Where are these cells destroyed?

10.7 List four events in a pregnancy that may be associated with a significant fetomaternal haemorrhage.

Guy's Hospital		Surname	F
Department of Blood Transfusion		Forename	H
Date 10.10.06		Sex	F
		DOB	11.11.82
		Number	731111
Blood Group	A Rhesus Negative		
Atypical Antibodies	Present		
Specificity	Anti-D Antibodies		
Quantitation	8 i.u./ml		

11.1   What is the illustrated instrument used for?

11.2   Name two important contraindications.

11.3   Where is the transcutaneous electrical nerve stimulation (TENS) placed? Name two sites.

11.4   Name two side-effects of nitrous oxide.

11.5   What is the most serious maternal side-effect of pethidine?

11.6   Why should pethidine not be used in fulminating pre-eclampsia?

11.7   What nerve roots does the pudendal nerve arise from?

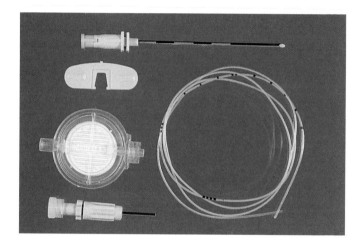

12.1   What is shown in this photograph?

12.2   Name four features that are normal.

12.3   If a fetus is distressed, what features would you expect? Name three.

12.4   In labour, how else can fetal well-being be assessed? Name two methods.

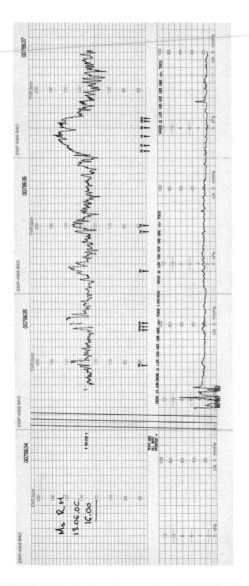

This baby is 2 days old and was 4.8 kg at birth.

13.1 What is the term used to describe this baby?

13.2 How may this have been detected antenatally. Name two methods.

13.3 What problem may have occurred in labour?

13.4 What problem may have occurred at delivery?

13.5 What problems may the baby develop neonatally? Name four.

13.6 Where should the baby be cared for during the first 24 hours?

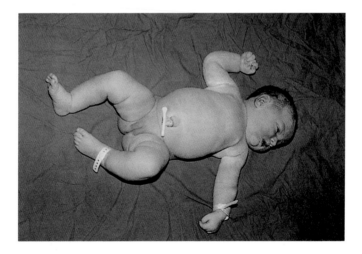

The specimen shown was obtained from a 66-year-old woman.

14.1 What is the most likely symptom that she may have presented with?

14.2 Name three risk factors for this condition.

14.3 What is the most likely histological diagnosis?

14.4 What is the premalignant phase histologically?

14.5 Where does it usually spread to? Name two sites.

14.6 What is the treatment for early stage disease?

14.7 What is the 5-year survival for stage 1 disease?

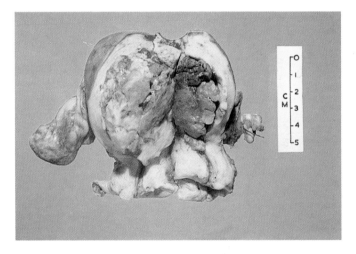

Miss TD is 17 years old and has had 11 weeks of amenorrhoea. For the last 3 weeks she has complained of nausea and vomiting and she has had heavy vaginal bleeding for 2 days.

15.1 An ultrasound has been performed. What does this show?

15.2 What does this appearance suggest?

15.3 What is the prevalence of this condition in the UK?

15.4 List two predisposing factors for this condition.

15.5 Which hormonal assay is useful in the management of this condition?

15.6 What is the treatment?

15.7 Histology confirms your diagnosis. How would you follow up Miss TD? Specify the test, where this should be performed, the frequency and the duration.

15.8 What is the usual method of treating chorion carcinoma?

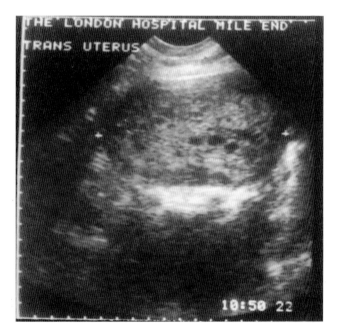

Mrs OT is 23 years old and presents to accident and emergency with a 6-hour history of constant right iliac fossa pain with intermittent gripping exacerbations. She has vomited on four occasions when the pain was at its worst. Her temperature is 37°C, there is guarding and rebound tenderness in the lower abdomen and she has marked tenderness in the right fornix. Her full blood count and transvaginal ultrasound report are shown.

16.1 What is the likely diagnosis?

16.2 List three important differential diagnoses.

16.3 What is the definitive investigation?

16.4 How soon should this investigation be performed? Explain why.

16.5 You confirm your diagnosis with your definitive investigation. Describe the principles of surgical management. Specify three.

Guy's Hospital **Department of Haematology**	Surname _____ T _____ Forename _____ O _____
Date 12.12.06	Sex _____ F _____ DOB _____ 12.11.83 _____ Number _____ 741112 _____

Haemoglobin   12.5 g/dl
White cell count $17.6 \times 10^9/l$
Platelet count $199 \times 10^{12}/l$

Guy's Hospital **Department of Radiology**	Surname _____ T _____ Forename _____ O _____
Date 12.12.06	Sex _____ F _____ DOB _____ 12.11.83 _____ Number _____ 741112 _____

Transvaginal ultrasound report

The uterus is anteverted and measures 12×5 cm^2.
A midline echo is seen.
The left ovary measures $3 \times 2.8 \times 4$ cm^3.
A 7-cm cystic area of mixed echogenicity is seen on the right and appears to arise from the right ovary.
Free fluid is seen in the peritoneal cavity.
Note: marked discomfort on introducing probe, particularly on the right.

This 44-year-old woman presented to the clinic complaining of regular heavy periods for 2 years. Her FBC is illustrated.

17.1   What is the normal blood loss per menstruation?

17.2   Name two terms to describe this woman's anaemia.

17.3   In the outpatient department, what would you do? Name three courses of action.

17.4   Name four medical treatments for menorrhagia.

Guy's Hospital **Department of Haematology**		Surname	P
		Forename	H
Date 2.11.06		Sex	F
		DOB	19.10.62
		Number	521019
Haemoglobin	7.6 g/dl		
White cell count	$11.1 \times 10^9/l$		
Platelet count	$247 \times 10^{12}/l$		
MCV	76 fl		
PCV	39%		
MCH	25 pg		
MCHC	27 g/dl		

This illustration shows a laparoscopic colposuspension being performed.

18.1 What is the medium used to distend the peritoneal cavity/cave of Retzius?

18.2 Name three complications that can occur on insertion of the trocar.

18.3 Name two safety measures performed prior to commencing laparoscopic surgery.

18.4 Name two advantages of a laparoscopic procedure over an open procedure for this patient.

18.5 What must the patient be prepared to accept when embarking upon any laparoscopic procedure?

18.6 If a patient complains of shoulder tip pain after a laparoscopy, what is the most likely cause?

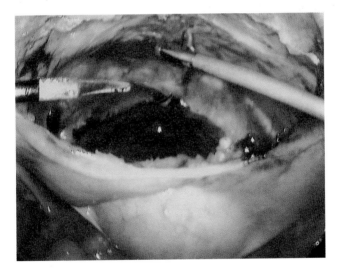

These laparoscopic views were obtained from a woman who presented with pelvic pain.

19.1 What is the diagnosis?

19.2 Name two signs you may have found on pelvic examination in the outpatient clinic.

19.3 Name three theories of the pathogenesis of this disease.

19.4 Name three medical treatments.

19.5 What is the incidence of this disease?

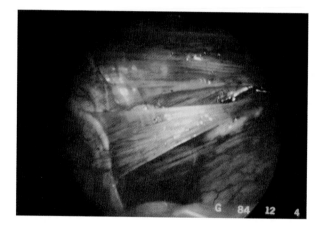

A

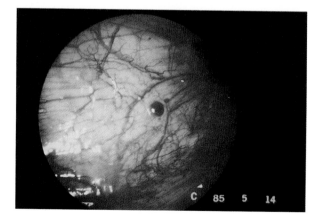

B

This woman presented with IMB.

20.1 What operation is being performed?

20.2 What can you see?

20.3 What management is indicated?

20.4 What other causes are there for IMB? Name three.

20.5 What media can be used to distend the cavity? Name two.

20.6 Is the histology likely to be benign or malignant?

20.7 How else might this problem have been diagnosed?

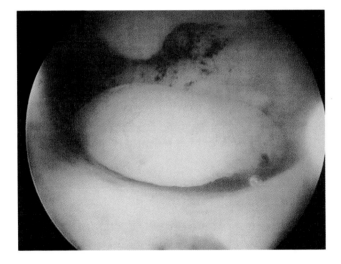

1.1   Ortolani's manoeuvre (test) [Marks 1]

1.2   Limited abduction of the hip, clunk or click during active abduction [Marks 2]

1.3   Congenital dislocation of the hip [Marks 1]

1.4   1–2/1000 births [Marks 1]

1.5   10–15% [Marks 1]

1.6   Yes; girls are more commonly affected than boys (6:1) [Marks 1]

1.7   Extended breech presentation [Marks 1]

1.8   Orthopaedic surgeon/paediatric orthopaedic surgeon [Marks 1]

1.9   Abduction splint (Von Rosen splint) [Marks 1]

2.1   Filschie clip [Marks 1]

2.2   Occludes the tube [Marks 1]

2.3   Hulka clip, fallope ring [Marks 2]

2.4   Sterilisation/laparoscopic sterilisation [Marks 1]

2.5   1 in 200 to 1 in 500 [Marks 1]

2.6   Permanent procedure, failure rate [Marks 2]

2.7   Clip applied to wrong structure, incomplete application of clip to fallopian tube [Marks 2]

3.1   Adhesions between the liver and the diaphragm [Marks 1]

3.2   Fitz-Hugh Curtis syndrome [Marks 1]

3.3   Chlamydia [Marks 1]

3.4 Endocervical swab [Marks 1]

3.5 Doxycycline, erythromycin [Marks 2]

3.6 Conjunctivitis [Marks 1]

3.7 Non-specific urethritis (NSU) [Marks 1]

3.8 Gonorrhoea [Marks 1]

3.9 Penicillin [Marks 1]

Station 4   ANSWERS   Circuit D

4.1 National Confidential Enquiry into Patient Outcome and Death [Marks 1]

4.2 1988 [Marks 1]

4.3 Previously National Confidential Enquiry into Peri-operative Deaths [Marks 1]

4.4 Deaths occurring in hospital within 30 days of surgery [Marks 2]

4.5 40% [Marks 1]

4.6 4.5% (accept 4–4.5%) [Marks 1]

4.7 20.1% [Marks 1]

4.8 59.2% [Marks 1]

4.9 Increase in senior trainee/trained surgeons' input from 31 to 59% at night. Almost 100% improvement [Marks 1]

Station 5   ANSWERS   Circuit D

5.1 Protein [Marks 1]

5.2 >5 g/l [Marks 1]

5.3 FBC and platelets, U&E, urate, 24-hour urine, clotting studies, liver enzymes [Marks 5]

5.4 Admit to hospital [Marks 1]

5.5 Pre-eclampsia, renal disease [Marks 2]

6.1 Pulling on the cord without suprapubic counter-traction to stop uterus inverting, morbid adherence of the placenta [Marks 2]

6.2 Manually reverse inversion immediately [Marks 1]

6.3 Hydrostatic method/O'Sullivan's method [Marks 1]

6.4 Manual removal was unsuccessful and therefore laparotomy was performed, ending in hysterectomy, massive haemorrhage [Marks 1]

6.5 Massive haemorrhage, DIC, anaesthetic complications, damage to other structures, e.g. ureter, bladder [Marks 3]

6.6 No [Marks 1]

6.7 Implantation in the lower segment, previous uterine scar [Marks 1]

7.1 Sickle cell trait [Marks 1]

7.2 Mrs AS's partner [Marks 1]

7.3 1:4, 1:2, 1:4 [Marks 3]

7.4 Fetal blood sampling and analysis of globin synthesis genes [Marks 2]

7.5 18–20 weeks [Marks 1]

7.6 Amniotic fluid fibroblasts/amniocentesis, chorion villus biopsy [Marks 2]

8.1 Engorged (swollen) with erythema [Marks 1]

8.2 Mastitis [Marks 1]

8.3 *Staphylococcus aureus* [Marks 1]

8.4 Oral flucloxacillin 250 mg QDS, oral erythromycin 250 mg QDS (in those allergic to penicillin) [Marks 1]

8.5 Incomplete emptying of breasts/milk stasis, and cracked or traumatised nipples [Marks 2]

8.6 Discontinue feeding from the affected breast; express manually from the affected breasts [Marks 2]

8.7 Breast abscess [Marks 1]

8.8 Incision and drainage [Marks 1]

| Station 9 | ANSWERS | Circuit D |

9.1 Intrauterine gestation sac, singleton fetus [Marks 2]

9.2 Crown rump length [Marks 1]

9.3 24 mm (approximately equal to 9 weeks and 2 days of gestation) [Marks 2]

9.4 Missed abortion [Marks 1]

9.5 Full blood count, group and save [Marks 2]

9.6 Evacuation of retained products of conception, general anaesthetic [Marks 2]

| Station 10 | ANSWERS | Circuit D |

10.1 Abnormally high level of anti-D antibody [Marks 1]

10.2 17% (accept 15–20%) [Marks 1]

10.3 Haemolytic disease of the newborn/haemolytic anaemia/hydrops fetalis [Marks 1]

10.4 Maternal IgG [Marks 1]

10.5 Fetal red cell D antigen [Marks 1]

10.6 Fetal spleen [Marks 1]

10.7 Miscarriage/bleeding in early pregnancy, ectopic pregnancy, amniocentesis/CVS/cordocentesis, APH, delivery, abdominal trauma [Marks 4]

11.1 Epidural [Marks 1]

11.2 Coagulopathy, sepsis, fixed output state [Marks 2]

11.3 Over the posterior primary rami of T10–L1 and S2–S4 [Marks 2]

11.4 Light-headedness, nausea [Marks 2]

11.5 Delaying gastric emptying [Marks 1]

11.6 Because the major metabolite has convulsant properties [Marks 1]

11.7 S2, S3, S4 [Marks 1]

12.1 A cardiotocograph [Marks 1]

12.2 Fetal heart rate of 140/min, good variability of >15 beats/min, accelerations, fetal movement [Marks 4]

12.3 Decelerations, tachycardia, bradycardia, loss of variability [Marks 3]

12.4 Liquor colour, fetal blood sample, umblical artery Doppler studies [Marks 2]

13.1 Macrosomia [Marks 1]

13.2 Measuring symphysiofundal height, USS measurements [Marks 2]

13.3 Failure to progress [Marks 1]

13.4 Shoulder dystocia [Marks 1]

13.5 Hypoglycaemia, hyperbilirubinaemia, hypocalcaemia, respiratory distress syndrome, fitting/convulsions [Marks 4]

13.6 In the special care baby unit [Marks 1]

14.1 Postmenopausal bleeding [Marks 1]

14.2 Obesity, polycystic ovarian syndrome (PCOS), nulliparity, late menopause, diabetes mellitus, unopposed oestrogen therapy [Marks 3]

14.3 Adenocarcinoma [Marks 1]

14.4 Endometrial hyperplasia with atypia [Marks 1]

14.5 Myometrium, pelvic lymph nodes, para-aortic nodes [Marks 2]

14.6 Total abdominal hysterectomy and bilateral salpingo-oopherectomy [Marks 1]

14.7 75% (70–80%) [Marks 1]

15.1 The appearance of vesicles [Marks 1]

15.2 Hydatidiform mole [Marks 1]

15.3 Approximately 1 in 1000 pregnancies [Marks 1]

15.4 Extremes of reproductive age (<15 or >45 years), south-east Asian origin, blood groups AB or BB [Marks 2]

15.5 Human chorionic gonadotrophin (urine or serum) [Marks 1]

15.6 Suction evacuation of the uterus [Marks 1]

15.7 Urinary BHCG sent to a supraregional centre at fortnightly intervals for 6 months to 2 years [Marks 2]

15.8 Chemotherapy/methotrexate [Marks 1]

16.1 Ovarian torsion [Marks 1]

16.2 Ectopic pregnancy, ovarian cyst haemorrhage (rupture), appendicitis/PID [Marks 3]

16.3 Laparoscopy [Marks 1]

16.4 Immediately. Delay will lead to ovarian necrosis/irreversible damage [Marks 2]

16.5 Untwist the ovarian pedicle. If the ovarian tissue looks viable, perform an ovarian cystectomy and conserve the ovary. If the ovary looks non-viable, remove the ovary [Marks 3]

| Station **17** | ANSWERS | Circuit **D** |

17.1 Less than 80 ml [Marks 1]

17.2 Microcytic, hypochromic [Marks 2]

17.3 History, pelvic examination, endometrial biopsy/hysteroscopy, smear if needed, transvaginal ultrasound (TVS) [Marks 3]

17.4 Antifibrinolytics, NSAID/mefenamic acid, COC pill, progestogens, progestogen-containing IUCD, LHRH analogues, danazol [Marks 4]

| Station **18** | ANSWERS | Circuit **D** |

18.1 CO_2 [Marks 1]

18.2 Haemorrhage (inferior epigastric, iliac vessel); perforation of a viscus (bowel, bladder); failure to enter peritoneal cavity [Marks 3]

18.3 Diathermy pad on patient, empty bladder, check gas flow, check equipment [Marks 2]

18.4 Shorter hospital stay, back to work quicker/back to normal activity, better cosmesis [Marks 2]

18.5 That a laparotomy may be needed [Marks 1]

18.6 CO_2 or blood irritating the diaphragm and causing referred pain to the shoulder tip [Marks 1]

19.1 Endometriosis [Marks 1]

19.2 A fixed retroverted uterus, tender uterosacral ligaments with nodules [Marks 2]

19.3 Coelomic metaplasia, retrograde menstruation, lymphatic/vascular spread, immunological reaction [Marks 3]

19.4 Continuous COC pill, danazol, GnRH analogues, progestogens (high dose), gestrinone [Marks 3]

19.5 10–40% [Marks 1]

20.1 Hysteroscopy [Marks 1]

20.2 Endometrial polyp [Marks 1]

20.3 Removal of the polyp [Marks 1]

20.4 Cervical polyp/cervical abnormality/cervical carcinoma, endometrial hyperplasia, endometrial carcinoma, hormone therapy, submucous fibroid [Marks 3]

20.5 Normal saline, glycine, CO_2 [Marks 2]

20.6 Benign [Marks 1]

20.7 Transvaginal scan [Marks 1]

Communication and Structured Oral Stations (CSOSs)

As this is a textbook rather than a live interactive situation, the demonstration of clinical and communication skills and structured oral stations is limited. The following examples will give you some idea as to what to expect. Prior to a communication station or structured oral station, there may be a rest station where information will be given to you for the actual communication/structured oral station. This will give you time to prepare for the encounter.

Remember that at the communication stations, communication is being assessed and knowledge is often secondary. The purpose of these stations is to assess your ability to communicate with the patients, so you must always treat them as individuals and be considerate. You want to convey to the examiner that you are a kind, compassionate and discerning clinician. As soon as you arrive at this station introduce yourself to the patient or the role-player. Remember that some patients are excellent historians and some are not. The role-player may have been briefed not to communicate well and therefore the station is assessing your skill to extract information. If there is a role-player at the station, she will have been briefed to give the same scenario to each candidate. The marking system will not be given to you and be aware that the role-player or patient may be awarding some marks.

With regard to structured orals, this scenario will involve yourself and the examiner. In some cases, the examiner may be role-playing, e.g. as a general practitioner, or may merely be asking you questions. There should be a logical flow to the structured oral. Whatever answer you give, the examiner may be instructed to present the contrary view. The following are examples of communication stations and structured orals.

Previous rest station – instructions to candidate

At the next station you will meet Mrs RT. She is a 34-year-old primigravida and she is currently at 37 weeks gestation. You need to check her BP, examine her abdomen and check for oedema.

Marking scheme	Marks
1. Introduction	1
2. Taking BP correctly (positioning etc.) and getting the correct BP	1
3. Observing the abdomen and detecting the laparoscopy scar	1
4. Measuring symphysiofundal height	1
5. Assessing presentation	1
6. Determining engagement of the head	1
7. Determining lie	1
8. Testing for oedema adequately	1

Marks from patient

1. Rapport	1
2. Not hurting patient during examination	1

Instructions to role-player

You have had pelvic pain premenstrually for 3 years. One year ago when you were in the States you had a laparoscopy and were told you had endometriosis. You did not attend for follow-up. Now you have come to see your GP/gynaecologist for an explanation about the disease and what treatments are available. Embarrassingly, you have recently noticed pain with intercourse and you suspect this may be related to endometriosis. You want to discuss endometriosis with the GP/gynaecologist and would like to bring up the problem with intercourse if he/she makes you feel comfortable enough.

Instructions to candidate

Your next patient has just booked under your care and has come for her first consultation.

Marking scheme	Marks
1. Introduction	1
2. Good rapport	1
3. Explaining the disease in easy terms	1
4. Being sympathetic	1
5. Explaining the options coherently	1
6. Extracting embarrassing problem	1

Marks from role-player

1. Felt confidence in candidate	1
2. Candidate gave good explanations	1
3. Would like to see him/her again	1
4. Candidate allowed role-player to choose between treatment options	1

Rest station – instructions to candidate

You are the SHO on call and you are about to take a phone call from a GP. When you arrive at the next station, pick up the telephone and speak to the GP.

Information to GP/examiner

You are a medical registrar and you know very little about gynaecology. You are doing a GP locum and a woman has arrived in your surgery with a history of unprotected intercourse 18 hours ago. You have no idea what to do, so rather embarrassingly you have rung the SHO on call in gynaecology. You want to find out what to do, when to do it and what the follow-up should be. You have heard that this certain SHO is rather arrogant so you are slightly on the defensive.

Marking scheme	Marks
1. Introduction	1
2. Finding out what the problem is	1
3. Finding out when intercourse occurred	1
4. Being sympathetic to the GP's lack of knowledge regarding postcoital contraception	1
5. Clearly describing how to take the appropriate tablets	1
6. Discussing insertion IUCD	1
7. Checking that the GP has understood	1
8. Was the SHO overall easy to understand?	1
9. Was it obvious that the SHO knew what he was talking about?	1
10. Would you be happy to call this SHO about a problem again?	1

Information to candidate

You are the SHO on call. You receive a call from a local GP. He has been to see a 41-year-old nulliparous woman who has a 12-month history of very heavy irregular periods and on this occasion she is soaking a pad every 30 minutes and this has been occurring for 8 hours. He has telephoned you and wants you to admit the patient, but you feel you can handle it by giving telephone advice.

Instructions to local GP

Scenario as above. You want her admitted.

Marking scheme

	Marks
1. SHO introducing himself on telephone	1
2. Being sympathetic to the GP's problem (woman distressed as bleeding at home)	1
3. Firmly refusing admission	1
4. Giving advice to stop bleeding – high-dose progestogens	1
5. Advising the GP to check haemoglobin	1
6. Advising the GP to give iron	1
7. Arranging outpatient appointment	1
8. Reassuring the GP	1
9. Indicating what will happen in OP	1
10. Telling the GP to call back if he has further concerns	1

Information to candidate

A midwife has just seen Mrs RT at home. She is 39 weeks pregnant and complains of reduced fetal movements. The midwife has arranged a CTG which is shown to you as illustrated. Ask the midwife about any other information you think may be relevant and advise her regarding further management.

Information to midwife

Mrs RT is a 22-year-old primigravida at 39 weeks gestation. She is a healthy non-smoker and her antenatal course has been completely uneventful so far. Today she says the baby is not moving as much. Her blood pressure is 110/80 mmHg with no proteinuria and the baby appears clinically to be well grown with adequate liquor. You are not convinced that the CTG is abnormal enough to warrant intervention but have come to ask the doctor's opinion.

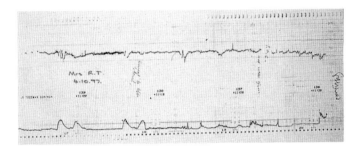

Marking scheme

	Marks
1. Courteous and polite approach	1
2. Listening to the midwife	1
3. Obtaining other relevant history	1
4. Explaining that the CTG is abnormal and that the fetus should be delivered	1
5. Avoiding confrontational exchange	1
6. Giving clear instructions without appearing condescending	1
7. Asking the midwife if she has questions	1
8. Following verbal and non-verbal clues	1

Marks from midwife

1. Confidence in the candidate's advice	1
2. Candidate was not antagonistic	1

Information to candidate

A community midwife comes to see you. She has seen Mrs EC, a 23-year-old primigravida at 32 weeks gestation, at home. Her booking blood pressure at 12 weeks was 110/60 mmHg and today it was 140/90 mmHg with + proteinuria. She asks your advice regarding further management.

Information to midwife

You have been to see Mrs EC at home. She is a 23-year-old healthy, non-smoking primigravida. She is 32 weeks pregnant with occasional headaches and she has noticed swelling of the fingers over the last 2 weeks. On examination, her blood pressure is 140/90 mmHg with + proteinuria. Abdominal examination reveals a symphysiofundal height of 26 cm, the presentation is cephalic and the fetus is active. You would like to manage the patient at home if possible.

Marking scheme   Marks

	Marks
1. Courteous and polite approach	1
2. Listening to the midwife	1
3. Obtaining other relevant information	1
4. Reassuring the midwife that the patient can be managed as an outpatient	1
5. Giving clear instructions regarding which investigations should be arranged	1
6. Giving clear instructions regarding indications for admission	1
7. Asking the midwife if she has any questions	1
8. Following verbal and non-verbal clues	1

Marks from midwife

1. Confidence in the candidate's advice	1
2. Rapport with the candidate	1

Information to candidate

Mrs AD is 43 years old and presents to your antenatal clinic at 10 weeks gestation in her second pregnancy. Her first pregnancy 2 years ago ended in miscarriage at 9 weeks. Her midwife has sent her to you to discuss antenatal diagnosis of congenital abnormalities. Counsel her regarding indications for antenatal tests and which tests are available.

Information to role-player

You are a very anxious 43-year-old and are worried about another miscarriage. You want as little interference with the pregnancy as possible and even if your baby had a congenital abnormality you would want to keep your baby. You are convinced that you will be forced to have an amniocentesis which will put your pregnancy at risk. During the consultation, ask these two specific questions:

- *Do I have to have an amniocentesis?*
- *Can't you see if the baby is alright on scan?*

Marking scheme	Marks
1. Introduction	1
2. Putting the patient at ease	1
3. Appropriate 'eye' contact	1
4. Listening to the patient	1
5. Extracting appropriate information	1
— wants little interference	
— would not terminate fetus	
6. Asking the patient if she has any questions	1
7. Reassuring that amniocentesis is not compulsory	1
8. Explaining that USS will pick up gross abnormalities but that chromosomal anomalies may be missed	1

Marks from role-player	
1. Confidence in the candidate	1
2. Rapport	1

Information to candidate

Mrs TO is 29 years old and has a 7-year-old son from her previous marriage. She and her current partner have been trying to conceive for 2½ years without success. Take a history from Mrs TO and explain the initial tests you are going to arrange – hormone profile and semen analysis.

Information to role-player

You are very anxious about not being able to have a baby. You stopped taking combined oral contraception 3 years ago and since then your periods have become very infrequent. In the last 6 months you have noticed a white discharge from the nipples. Do not offer this information unless specifically asked.

Your last menstrual period was 6 months ago. Your current partner is 26 and has two children from a previous marriage.

Marking scheme	Marks
1. Introduction	1
2. Putting the patient at ease	1
3. Appropriate 'eye' contact	1
4. Listening to the patient	1
5. Extracting appropriate information (amenorrhoea, galactorrhoea)	1
6. Explaining hormone profile	1
7. Explaining semen analysis	1
8. Asking if the patient has any questions	1

Marks from role-player

1. Confidence in the candidate	1
2. Rapport	1

1.1 The examiner has three pairs of forceps in front of him/her, as shown in the photograph. Name the three forceps illustrated from top to bottom.

1.2 The examiner describes the following scenario: 'A woman has been pushing in the second stage for 2 hours and is exhausted; there is no head palpable abdominally and the head is at station +2, direct occipito-anterior'. Which forceps would you use?

1.3 The examiner says, 'Having decided to deliver by forceps, what type of analgesia could you use?'. Name two.

1.4 Before applying the forceps, what other requirements must you ensure have been met? Name two.

1.5 The examiner picks up the middle and lower forceps and asks you to name two differences between them.

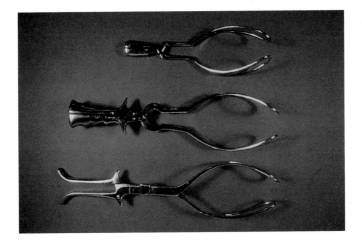

Rest station
Read the histology report below. The examiner at the next station will ask you some questions about it.

2.1   What procedure has been performed?

2.2   Describe the procedure.

2.3   The procedure was performed in colposcopy clinic. What anaesthetic would you have used?

2.4   Describe how you would carry out this procedure and what you would use.

2.5   Name two late complications of this procedure.

2.6   What further treatment would you suggest? Name two aspects.

Histology Report
Specimen measures $2.8 \times 2.4 \times 1.6$ cm^3
The whole specimen has been processed. At the squamocolumnar junction there is extensive full-thickness cervical intraepithelial neoplasia III. The lesion appears to extend to the endocervical margins of excision, although this is difficult to determine as there is diathermy damage. There is no evidence of invasion.

Summary
CIN III, which may be incompletely excised. No evidence of invasion.

3.1 Describe the components shown in the box. Name four.

3.2 What is the appliance shown?

3.3 In general terms, after what type of surgical procedure is this appliance usually used?

3.4 What is the commonest complication of inserting such an appliance?

3.5 If this is suspected, what investigation is indicated?

3.6 If this complication is confirmed, which two measures should you aim to undertake?

Note: In the live situation, this question could involve you demonstrating catheter insertion on a pelvic model.

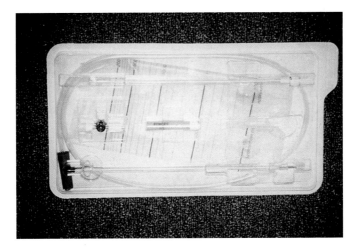

You are provided with a model of a fetal skull and female pelvis.

4.1   Demonstrate and describe the mechanism of normal labour.

4.2   Demonstrate:
1. **Deep transverse arrest**
2. **Occipitoposterior position**
3. **Brow presentation**
4. **Face presentation**

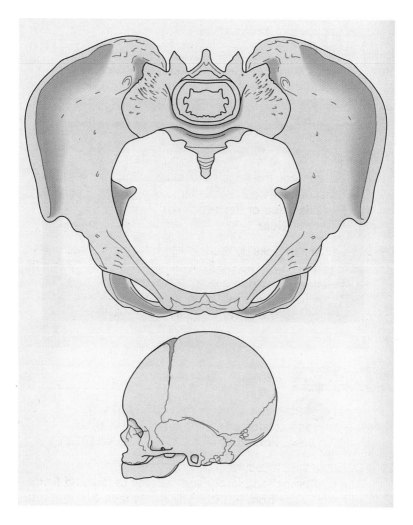

1.1 Wrigley's, Neville–Barnes/Anderson's/Simpson's, Kielland's [Marks 3]

1.2 Neville–Barnes (the middle one) [Marks 1]

1.3 Epidural, spinal, pudendal [Marks 2]

1.4 Full dilatation of the cervix, empty bladder [Marks 2]

1.5 The lower one has a sliding lock. The middle one has both a cephalic and a pelvic curve, and the lower one has no pelvic curve [Marks 2]

2.1 Large loop excision of the transformation zone (LLETZ)/laser cone/ diathermy loop excision (DLE) [Marks 1]

2.2 The diathermy loop is passed into the cervix and from right to left or from left to right and is then brought out. The specimen resembles a cone [Marks 2]

2.3 Paracervical block [Marks 1]

2.4 Infiltrate at 3, 6, 9, 12 o'clock with an adrenalin-containing local anaesthetic [Marks 2]

2.5 Infertility, cervical stenosis, cervical incompetence [Marks 2]

2.6 Follow-up smears, repeat diathermy loop excision/cone biopsy, hysterectomy [Marks 2]

3.1 Three-way tap, catheter connector, catheter, catheter bag [Marks 4]

3.2 A suprapubic catheter (SPC) [Marks 1]

3.3 Surgery to stabilise bladder neck/surgery for genuine stress incontinence [Marks 1]

3.4 Urinary tract infection [Marks 1]

3.5 CSU for microscopy/culture and sensitivity [Marks 1]

3.6 Remove SPC as soon as practicable, treat with appropriate antibiotics [Marks 2]

4.1 One mark each is given for:
1. Engagement
2. Flexion
3. Internal rotation
4. Descent
5. Extension
6. Restitution

One mark each is given for demonstrating and describing:
1. Deep transverse arrest
2. Occipitoposterior position
3. Brow presentation
4. Face presentation [Marks 10]

Extended Matching Questions (EMQs)

1) Gynaecology Procedures

A. Vaginal hysterectomy
B. Large loop excision of the transformation zone (LLETZ)
C. Colposuspension
D. Colposcopy
E. Hysteroscopy
F. Hysteroscopic resection of fibroid/polyp
G. Laparoscopy
H. Anterior vaginal repair
I. Posterior vaginal repair
J. Tension free vaginal tape
K. Total abdominal hysterectomy
L. Endometrial ablation
M. Laparoscopic sterilisation
N. Manchester repair
O. Progestogen IUS

For each of the scenarios below choose the most appropriate procedure from the list above. Each procedure may be used once, more than once or not at all.

1. A 52-year-old woman has a 5-year history of menorrhagia and an 18-week size fibroid uterus causing significant pressure symptoms.

2. A 45-year-old woman has a 6-month history of heavy regular periods and intermenstrual bleeding. A transvaginal ultrasound scan shows an endometrial thickness of 16 mm and appearances suggestive of an endometrial polyp.

3. A 34-year-old multiparous woman has her routine smear result, which shows moderate dyskaryosis.

4. A 62-year-old woman complains of urinary incontinence with laughing and coughing but no urinary frequency. Examination reveals a cystocoele with no growth on midstream urine culture. The urodynamic studies show evidence of stress incontinence.

5. A 40-year-old woman presents with worsening menorraghia. A transvaginal ultrasound scan shows normal appearances of the uterus and ovaries. Pipelle biopsy shows proliferative endometrium. She does not want an operation.

6. A 26-year-old woman presents with painful periods and dyspareunia On examination she has a fixed retroverted uterus.

7. A 60-year-old woman has a feeling of 'something coming down' into her vagina. She has a feeling of incomplete emptying with micturition but no bowel symptoms. Examination reveals uterine descent.

8. A 28-year-old woman wants effective contraception after having four normal deliveries. She currently has no stable partner.

2) Drugs in Pregnancy

    A. Premature closure of Ductus Arteriosus
    B. Skull defects
    C. Growth restriction
    D. Limb defects
    E. Dental discoloration
    F. 8th cranial nerve damage
    G. Neural tube defects
    H. Myelosuppression

For each of the drugs below, select the most appropriate unwanted effect from the list above. Each unwanted effect may be selected once, more than once or not at all.

1. Aminoglycosides

2. Beta blockers

3. Thalidomide

4. Tetracyclines in late pregnancy

5. Non-steroidal anti-inflammatory drugs if given in late pregnancy

6. Sodium valproate

7. Angiotensin converting enzyme inhibitors

8. Azathioprine

3) Hormone Profiles

    A. Low FSH and LH, low oestradiol
    B. High FSH and LH, low oestradiol
    C. High LH/FSH ratio
    D. Low FSH and LH, high oestradiol
    E. High FSH and LH, high oestradiol

For each of the clinical presentations below, select the most appropriate hormone profile from the list above.

1. Ovarian failure

2. Marathon runner

3. PCOS

4. Oestrogen secreting tumour

5. Anorexia nervosa

6. Ovulation

4) Maternal Systemic Disorders in Pregnancy

A. DVT
B. Iron deficiency
C. Antiphospholipid syndrome
D. Diabetes mellitus
E. Impaired glucose tolerance
F. Folate deficiency
G. Thrombocytopenia
H. Baker's cyst
J. Cholestasis of pregnancy
K. Twin pregnancy
L. Thrombophilia
M. Hepatitis
N. Sickle cell disease

Match the clinical scenario 1–8 with the most likely diagnosis from the list A–N.

1. A 32-year-old woman with a painful right calf that appears to be swollen and is tender.

2. A 30-year-old woman with raised liver function tests and bile acids and pruritus.

3. A pregnant woman who is tired, with a low MCV, MCH, MCHC and a haemoglobin concentration of 10.0 g/dl.

4. A pregnant woman who is tired, with a raised MCV and a haemoglobin concentration of 10.0 g/dl.

5. A woman with a 2-hour post 75-g oral glucose load serum glucose concentration of 9 mmol/l.

6. A woman with a 2-hour post 75-g oral glucose load serum glucose concentration of 11.4 mmol/l.

7. A woman with severe pre-eclampsia who has had one previous midtrimester miscarriage.

8. A woman who has a platelet count of 50×10^9.

5) Oligomenorrhoea, Infertility

    A. Weight loss
    B. Ovarian diathermy
    C. Oral clomifene therapy
    D. Oral cyproterone acetate therapy
    E. Free androgen index
    F. Glucose tolerance test
    G. Follicular tracking
    H. Transvaginal ultrasonography
    I. Mid-luteal serum progesterone assay
    J. Oral metformin therapy
    K. Serum prolactin
    L. Thyroid function tests
    M. Endometrial biopsy
    N. CA125
    O. Urinary beta HCG

For each of the scenarios below choose the single most appropriate intervention from the statements listed above. Each statement may be used once, more than once or not at all.

1. A 32-year-old nulliparous woman presents with no period for 10 weeks.

2. A 26-year-old woman has a 3-year-old child who she breastfed for 15 months. She has not menstruated since her delivery and has noticed continuing milky discharge from her breasts.

3. A 19-year-old woman reports not having a period for 6 months and is virgo intacta. She is very embarrassed because she has noticed dark hair around her nipples and navel.

4. A 29-year-old nulliparous woman and her partner have not used contraception for 18 months and have failed to conceive a child despite regular coitus. Her partner has a normal semen analysis.

5. A 22-year-old woman weighs 92 kg with a height of 1.55 m. She reports no periods for 9 months. She is not sexually active but is concerned about her lack of periods.

6. A 29-year-old woman with a BMI of 22 presenting with primary infertility has been diagnosed with PCOS. Her husband has a normal semen analysis.

7. A 40-year-old woman complains of tiredness and lethargy. On specific questioning she reports weight gain and infrequent periods.

8. A 44-year-old woman presents with weight loss and infrequent periods. On direct questioning she complains of excessive thirst and urinary frequency.

9. A 25-year-old woman with a BMI of 23 with primary infertility and PCOS has had 6 months of treatment with clomifene citrate 200 mg D2-6 but fails to ovulate.

10. During investigation of secondary amenorrhoea a 39-year-old woman is found to have the appearances of a multilocular 8 cm diameter cyst on pelvic ultrasound.

6) Ectopic Pregnancy

   A. 250 i.u. ANTI-D administered intramuscularly
   B. Endocervical swabs for M, C & S
   C. Resuscitation and laparotomy
   D. Medical management with systemic methotrexate
   E. Transfusion with type O negative blood
   F. Pelvic ultrasound
   G. Laparoscopy and salpingotomy
   H. Combined oral contraceptive
   I. Intrauterine device
   J. Two measurements of serum HCG 48 hours apart
   K. 14-day course of co-amoxyclav + doxycycline
   L. Hysterosalpingogram
   M. Barrier methods

**For each of the scenarios below choose the single most appropriate intervention from the statements listed.
Each statement may be used once, more than once or not at all.**

1. A 19-year-old woman arrives in A&E by ambulance. She is conscious with a blood pressure of 70/30 mmHg and pulse rate of 180/min. A catheter specimen of urine is positive for beta HCG.

2. A 24-year-old woman attends A&E with an 8-week history of amenorrhoea and bright red spotting. A urinary beta HCG is positive.

3. A 28-year-old woman with O rhesus-negative blood type presents with vaginal bleeding at 14 weeks gestation. The external cervical os is closed and the fetal heart is clearly audible with a Sonicaid.

4. A 35-year-old woman presents with a 7-week history of amenorrhoea, a positive pregnancy test and abdominal pain which is worse on the left. An ultrasound scan shows an empty uterus and a 2-cm-diameter mass close to the left ovary. She has had a previous salpingectomy for ectopic.

5. A 30-year-old woman arrives unconscious in A&E. She is extremely pale with a barely recordable blood pressure or pulse.

6. A 17-year-old woman presents with pelvic pain 5 weeks after her last period. She has been having unprotected coitus but a urine BHCG is negative. She has a mucopurulent vaginal discharge.

7. A transvaginal ultrasound scan in this woman shows an endometrial thickness of 20 mm but no gestation sac.

8. The same woman has worsening pain. A repeat scan 10 days after admission shows no intrauterine sac and small-volume free fluid in the pelvis. Serum HCG is approximately 1000 i.u./l but the patient adamantly refuses an operation.

9. A swab taken at admission is reported positive for Chlamydia antigen.

10. What would you advise this woman against re future contraception?

7) Pruritus in Pregnancy

    A. Treatment with ursodeoxycholic acid
    B. Serum alkaline phosphatase
    C. Serum transaminases, gamma glutamyl transferase, bile salts
    D. Viral screen for hepatitis A, B, C, CMV and EB
    E. Oral vitamin K 10 mg daily
    F. Elective caesarean section after 37 weeks gestation
    G. Induction of labour after 37 weeks gestation

H. Prothrombin time
I. Oral chlorpheniramine 4 mg 8-hourly
J. Oral dexamethasone 10 mg daily
K. Ultrasound scan of renal tract
L. 24-hour urinary protein excretion estimation
M. Induction of labour after 40 weeks gestation
N. Await spontaneous labour up to 41+5 weeks gestation

For each of the scenarios below choose the single most appropriate intervention from the statements listed. Each statement may be used once, more than once or not at all.

1. A 19-year-old primigravid woman attends the antenatal clinic at 33 weeks gestation complaining of intense itching of her hands and feet. Which first-line investigation(s) would you arrange?

2. Which other investigation(s) help in establishing the diagnosis?

3. The same woman complains that the itching is preventing her sleeping at night. What would you prescribe for symptomatic relief?

4. The woman has minimal relief from first-line treatment. What would you prescribe?

5. In some circumstances with severe refractory pruritus an alternative may relieve symptoms.

6. How would you aim to deliver this woman?

7. Two weeks after delivery her symptoms have completely subsided. How would you confirm your diagnosis?

8. You are concerned regarding an increased risk of post-partum haemorrhage. What would you recommend?

9. A 32-year-old woman with a history of cholestasis at 34 weeks in her previous pregnancy attends antenatal clinic at 36 weeks. She has a breech presentation and declines ECV. What would you advise?

10. A 19-year-old woman in her first pregnancy with serum aspartate transaminase of 70 i.u./l at 32 weeks develops 2+ proteinuria.

1) Gynaecology Procedures

For each of the scenarios below choose the most appropriate procedure from the list above. Each procedure may be used once, more than once or not at all.

1. A 52-year-old woman has a 5-year history of menorrhagia and an 18-week size fibroid uterus causing significant pressure symptoms.

   K. Total abdominal hysterectomy. A vaginal hysterectomy would not be appropriate in this case, as the uterus is so large. A laparotomy is needed to remove the uterus. If she wanted to keep her cervix, a subtotal hysterectomy would also be appropriate.

2. A 45-year-old woman has a 6-month history of heavy regular periods and intermenstrual bleeding. A transvaginal ultrasound scan shows an endometrial thickness of 16 mm and appearances suggestive of an endometrial polyp.

   F. Hysteroscopic resection of fibroid /polyp. The endometrial polyp is undoubtedly the cause of her intermenstrual bleeding and menorrhagia. Using the hysteroscope, the polyp can be resected under direct vision.

3. A 34-year-old multiparous woman has her routine smear result, which shows moderate dyskaryosis.

   D. Colposcopy. A smear of moderate dyskaryosis should always be referred for colposcopy.

4. A 62-year-old woman complains of urinary incontinence with laughing and coughing but no urinary frequency. Examination reveals a cystocoele with no growth on midstream urine culture. The urodynamic studies show evidence of stress incontinence.

   J. Tension free vaginal tape. This woman gives no history of urge incontinence and infection has been excluded. She therefore has pure stress incontinence and tension free vaginal tapes are used to elevate the urethra. A colposuspension would also be acceptable, but tension-free vaginal tapes are an easier operation and associated with less complications.

5. A 40-year-old woman presents with worsening menorrhagia. A transvaginal ultrasound scan shows normal appearances of the uterus and ovaries. Pipelle biopsy shows proliferative endometrium. She does not want an operation.

   O. Progestogen IUS. The Mirena Intrauterine System contains levonorgestrel and releases 20 µg a day, leading to a thinner endometrium or can even induce an atrophic endometrium. This, therefore, would improve her heavy bleeding and avoid an operation.

6. A 26-year-old woman presents with painful periods and dyspareunia. On examination she has a fixed retroverted uterus.

G. Laparoscopy. This is the classical history of a woman with endometriosis and the examination findings are in keeping with this. She needs a laparoscopy to make the diagnosis, assess the extent of the disease and, if endometriosis is present, it can be diathermied or excised at the same time.

7. A 60-year-old woman has a feeling of 'something coming down' into her vagina. She has a feeling of incomplete emptying with micturition but no bowel symptoms. Examination reveals uterine descent.

A. Vaginal hysterectomy. This woman has uterine prolapse, so a vaginal hysterectomy would be the best option for her. The feeling of incomplete emptying is probably due to the anatomical distortion that occurs when the bladder is pulled down with the uterus.

8. A 28-year-old woman wants effective contraception after having four normal deliveries. She currently has no stable partner.

O. Progestogen IUS. The Mirena Intrauterine System has a lower failure rate than laparoscopic sterilisation and has the added advantage of decreasing pelvic infection and decreasing menstrual flow. Even if she felt she had completed her family, it would be inadvisable to do a laparoscopic sterilisation, as she is only 28 and she is currently not in a stable relationship.

2) Drugs in Pregnancy

For each of the drugs below, select the most appropriate unwanted effect from the list above. Each unwanted effect may be selected once, more than once or not at all.

1. Aminoglycosides

F. 8th cranial nerve damage. All aminoglycosides cross the placenta and in utero-ototoxicity has been reported, with kanamycin and streptomycin, but not with amikacin, gentamicin, nor tobramycin.

2. Beta blockers

C. Growth restriction. Beta blockers are associated with intrauterine growth retardation when started in the second trimester.

3. Thalidomide

D. Limb defects. Thalidomide was mainly prescribed to pregnant women for morning sickness in the late 1950s and early 1960s. The drug caused severe deformities in babies with missing limbs.

4. Tetracyclines in late pregnancy

E. Dental discoloration. Tetracyclines exposure after the fourth month of pregnancy may result in brownish staining of the deciduous teeth. When administered near term, the permanent teeth may also be stained.

5. Non-steroidal anti-inflammatory drugs if given in late pregnancy

A. Premature closure of Ductus Arteriosus. Non-steriodal anti-inflammatory drugs used near term may cause premature closure of the ductus arteriosus and inhibit labour. Oligohydramnios after prolonged use is a common complication with NSAIDs as a class.

6. Sodium valproate

G. Neural tube defects. The incidence of neural tube defects (spina bifida) after first trimester exposure with sodium valproate is approximately 1%.

7. Angiotensin converting enzyme inhibitors

B. Skull defects. Use of ACE inhibitors in the second and third trimester is associated with hypocalvaria and renal defects related to fetal hypotension and decreased renal perfusion. The latter may result in oligohydramnios.

8. Azathioprine

H. Myelosuppression. Azathioprine is an anti-neoplastic.

3) Hormone Profiles

1. Ovarian failure

B. High FSH and LH, low oestradiol. As the ovaries start to fail, FSH and LH are raised to try and increase the output of oestrogen from the ovaries. However, when ovarian failure occurs, the ovary is unable to produce more oestrogen so the hormone profile has high gonadotrophins and a low oestradiol.

2. Marathon runner

  A. Low FSH and LH, low oestradiol. Women who exercise excessively switch off the HPO axis at the hypothalamus, so the pituitary is suppressed, resulting in ovarian suppression.

3. PCOS

  C. High LH/FSH ratio. In women with PCOS the LH/FSH ratio and serum oestradiol are raised. Testosterone and androstenedione are also characteristically elevated.

4. Oestrogen-secreting tumour

  D. Low FSH and LH, high oestradiol. With an oestrogen-secreting tumour, the oestradiol levels are high, therefore FSH and LH are low in response to the negative feedback at the pituitary level.

5. Anorexia nervosa

  A. Low FSH and LH, low oestradiol. As with women who exercise excessively, women with anorexia have cessation of function at the hypothalamic level.

6. Ovulation

  E. High FSH and LH, high oestradiol. At the time of ovulation oestradiol, FSH and LH are high.

4) Maternal Systemic Disorders in Pregnancy

1. A 32-year-old woman with a painful right calf that appears to be swollen and is tender.

  A. DVT. Pregnancy is a thrombogenic state and DVTs are common.

2. A 30-year-old woman with raised liver function tests and bile acids and pruritus.

  J. Cholestasis of pregnancy. Cholestasis of pregnancy is becoming a more common disorder and typically presents with pruritus and investigations will reveal raised liver function tests and bile acids.

3. A pregnant woman who is tired, with a low MCV, MCH, MCHC and a haemoglobin concentration of 10.0 g/dl.

  B. Iron deficiency. Pregnancy is draining on a woman's iron stores and iron deficiency anaemia is common.

4. A pregnant woman who is tired, with a raised MCV and a haemoglobin concentration of 10.0 g/dl.

  F. Folate deficiency. Vitamin B_{12} and folate deficiency present with hyperchromic anaemia.

5. A woman with a 2-hour post 75-g oral glucose load serum glucose concentration of 9 mmol/l.

   E. Impaired glucose tolerance. A glucose tolerance test (GTT) with a 75-g glucose load distinguishes between diabetes, impaired glucose tolerance and normality. Less than 7.8 mmol/l is normal, 7.8–11 mmol/l is impaired glucose tolerance and >11 mmol/l is gestational diabetes.

6. A woman with a 2-hour post 75-g oral glucose load serum glucose concentration of 11.4 mmol/l.

   D. Diabetes mellitus. Same as above.

7. A woman with severe pre-eclampsia who has had one previous midtrimester miscarriage.

   C. Antiphospholipid syndrome. The diagnosis of antiphospholipid syndrome depends on three first-trimester miscarriages, or one midtrimester or severe pre-eclampsia, IUGR or abruption, necessitating delivery prior to 37 weeks and the presence of anticardiolipin antibodies or lupus anticoagulant.

8. A woman who has a platelet count of 50×10^9.

   G. Thrombocytopenia. Up to 10% of women have a low platelet count in pregnancy, most commonly due to gestational thrombocytopenia. The platelet count decreases for most women throughout pregnancy and if it falls below 150×10^9 per litre, it is termed gestational thrombocytopenia.

5) Oligomenorrhoea, Infertility

1. A 32-year-old nulliparous woman presents with no period for 10 weeks.

   O. Urinary beta HCG. Pregnancy must be excluded in any woman of reproductive age presenting with secondary amenorrhoea.

2. A 26-year-old woman has a 3-year-old child who she breastfed for 15 months. She has not menstruated since her delivery and has noticed continuing milky discharge from her breasts.

   K. Serum prolactin. Prolactinoma must be considered in any woman of reproductive age presenting with amenorrhoea and galactorrhoea.

3. A 19-year-old woman reports not having a period for 6 months and is virgo intacta. She is very embarrassed because she has noticed dark hair around her nipples and navel.

E. Free androgen index. Hirsutism is one of the triad of features originally described in polycystic ovarian syndrome (PCOS). The most appropriate test from those listed is measurement of the ratio of serum testosterone to sex hormone binding globulin (free testosterone index).

4. A 29-year-old nulliparous woman and her partner have not used contraception for 18 months and have failed to conceive a child despite regular coitus. Her partner has a normal semen analysis.

   I. Mid-luteal serum progesterone assay. During the investigation of infertility it is paramount to establish whether the woman is ovulating. A mid-luteal progesterone assay is a simple test to check this.

5. A 22-year-old woman weighs 92 kg with a height of 1.55 m. She reports no periods for 9 months. She is not sexually active but is concerned about her lack of periods.

   H. Transvaginal ultrasonography. This woman with secondary amenorrhoea has a BMI of >38 kg/m^2. The likely diagnosis is PCOS which would usually produce a characteristic appearance of the ovaries on transvaginal ultrasonography.

6. A 29-year-old woman with a BMI of 22 presenting with primary infertility has been diagnosed with PCOS. Her husband has a normal semen analysis.

   C. Oral clomifene therapy. In cases of infertility associated with PCOS first-line treatment should be ovulation induction with clomifene after discussion of the risks of multiple pregnancy.

7. A 40-year-old woman complains of tiredness and lethargy. On specific questioning she reports weight gain and infrequent periods.

   L. Thyroid function tests. The symptoms described, although non-specific, are compatible with hypothyroidism which should be excluded.

8. A 44-year-old woman presents with weight loss and infrequent periods. On direct questioning she complains of excessive thirst and urinary frequency.

   F. Glucose tolerance test. The symptoms described are suggestive of diabetes mellitus which must be excluded.

9. A 25-year-old woman with a BMI of 23 with primary infertility and PCOS has had 6 months of treatment with clomifene citrate 200 mg D2-6 but fails to ovulate.

B. Ovarian diathermy. In cases of failed ovulation induction with clomifene the woman should be offered ovarian diathermy or laparoscopic ovarian drilling. Other options include combination treatment with clomifene and metformin.

10. During investigation of secondary amenorrhoea a 39-year-old woman is found to have the appearances of a multilocular 8-cm-diameter cyst on pelvic ultrasound.

N. CA125. Complex ovarian cysts should be investigated with serum CA125 to allow calculation of the risk of malignancy index (pertaining to epithelial ovarian tumours).

6) Ectopic Pregnancy

1. A 19-year-old woman arrives in A&E by ambulance. She is conscious with a blood pressure of 70/30 mmHg and pulse rate of 180/min. A catheter specimen of urine is positive for beta HCG.

C. Resuscitation and laparotomy. Unexplained hypotensive collapse in a woman of reproductive age group should arouse a high index of suspicion for ruptured ectopic pregnancy. If a pregnancy test is also positive the diagnosis is almost certain. Treatment is immediate resuscitation and exploratory laparotomy.

2. A 24-year-old woman attends A&E with an 8-week history of amenorrhoea and bright red spotting. A urinary beta HCG is positive.

F. Pelvic ultrasound. In any case of bleeding in early pregnancy the first-line investigation should be a pelvic ultrasound, preferably via the transvaginal route.

3. A 28-year-old woman with O rhesus-negative blood type presents with vaginal bleeding at 14 weeks gestation. The external cervical os is closed and the fetal heart is clearly audible with a Sonicaid.

A. 250 i.u. ANTI-D administered intramuscularly. Women with rhesus-negative blood group should be offered prophylaxis against rhesus isoimmunisation for any sensitising events after 12 weeks gestation.

4. A 35-year-old woman presents with a 7-week history of amenorrhoea, a positive pregnancy test and abdominal pain which is worse on the left. An ultrasound scan shows an empty uterus and a 2-cm-diameter mass close to the left ovary. She has had a previous salpingectomy for ectopic.

G. Laparoscopy and salpingotomy. The features described are of an ectopic pregnancy in a woman's only remaining tube. A laparoscopy and salpingotomy with conservation of the remaining tube should be attempted.

5. A 30-year-old woman arrives unconscious in A&E. She is extremely pale with a barely recordable blood pressure or pulse.

E. Transfusion with type O negative blood. In cases of profound hypotensive collapse immediate resuscitation with type O negative blood should be instituted as soon as the blood is available.

6. A 17-year-old woman presents with pelvic pain 5 weeks after her last period. She has been having unprotected coitus but a urine BHCG is negative. She has a mucopurulent vaginal discharge.

B. Endocervical swabs for MC&S. Any woman presenting with pelvic pain and a mucopurulent vaginal discharge should have endocervical swabs taken to exclude infection.

7. A transvaginal ultrasound scan in this woman shows an endometrial thickness of 20 mm but no gestation sac.

J. Two measurements of serum HCG 48 hours apart. Endometrial thickening may represent a decidual reaction. Serum HCG should be estimated on 2 occasions 48 hours apart.

8. The same woman has worsening pain. A repeat scan 10 days after admission shows no intrauterine sac and small-volume free fluid in the pelvis. Serum HCG is approximately 1000 i.u./l but the patient adamantly refuses an operation.

D. Medical management with systemic methotrexate.
The clinical features are indicative of a leaking ectopic pregnancy. If the patient refuses surgery she should be offered medical management with systemic methotrexate. Her response should be monitored with serial serum HCG measurements.

9. A swab taken at admission is reported positive for Chlamydia antigen.

K. 14-day course of co-amoxyclav + doxycycline. Chlamydia should be treated with doxycycline for 14 days or a single dose of azithromycin. Treatment is usually in combination with a broad spectrum antibiotic which covers anaerobic organisms. Appropriate contact tracing should be pursued which may require referral to the genitourinary medicine clinic.

10. What would you advise this woman against re future contraception?

  M. Barrier methods. After ectopic pregnancy an intrauterine device is relatively contraindicated. A number of options for contraception including barrier methods, the combined oral contraceptive and progesterone-only preparations are appropriate.

7) Pruritus in Pregnancy

1. A 19-year-old primigravid woman attends the antenatal clinic at 33 weeks gestation complaining of intense itching of her hands and feet. Which first-line investigation(s) would you arrange?

  C. Serum transaminases, gamma glutamyl transferase, bile salts. First-line investigation of pruritus in pregnancy should include serum transaminases, particularly alanine transaminase, and gamma glutamyl transferase. Bile salts are raised in almost all cases.

2. Which other investigation(s) help in establishing the diagnosis?

  D. Viral screen for hepatitis A, B, C, CMV and EB. Hepatitis serology to exclude viral hepatitis should be requested in all cases of suspected intrahepatic cholestasis of pregnancy (ICP).

3. The same woman complains that the itching is preventing her sleeping at night. What would you prescribe for symptomatic relief?

  I. Oral chlorpheniramine 4 mg 8-hourly. Antihistamines may give short-term relief of symptoms and improve sleep.

4. The woman has minimal relief from first-line treatment. What would you prescribe?

  A. Treatment with ursodeoxycholic acid. There is evidence that ursodeoxycholic acid, a natural hydrophilic bile salt, reduces pruritus as well as bile acid levels.

5. In some circumstances with severe refractory pruritus an alternative may relieve symptoms.

  J. Oral dexamethasone 10 mg daily. Pruritus is sometimes improved by treatment with oral dexamethasone.

6. How would you aim to deliver this woman?

  G. Induction of labour after 37 weeks gestation. The effect of maternal cholestasis on the unborn fetus is unpredictable. Several reports suggest higher stillbirth rates (up to 15%). Delivery should be considered as soon as the pregnancy reaches term and, in the absence of other obstetric indications, the vaginal route is preferred. In cases with rapidly rising transaminases and bile salts preterm elective delivery should be considered.

7. Two weeks after delivery her symptoms have completely subsided. How would you confirm your diagnosis?

   C. Serum transaminases, gamma glutamyl transferase, bile salts. In the majority of cases biochemical resolution occurs within 2 weeks of delivery. Ultrasonography of the biliary tract should be performed in all cases to exclude cholelithiasis.

8. You are concerned regarding an increased risk of post-partum haemorrhage. What would you recommend?

   E. Oral vitamin K 10 mg daily. There is a 10–20% risk of obstetric haemorrhage in cases of ICP attributable, in part, to vitamin K malabsorption. Vitamin K supplementation should be considered in all cases.

9. A 32-year-old woman with a history of cholestasis at 34 weeks in her previous pregnancy attends antenatal clinic at 36 weeks. She has a breech presentation and declines ECV. What would you advise?

   F. Elective caesarean section after 37 weeks gestation. As in question 6, delivery should be expedited but in this case there is an obstetric indication for elective caesarean section.

10. A 19-year-old woman in her first pregnancy with serum aspartate transaminase of 70 i.u./l at 32 weeks develops 2+ proteinuria.

   L. 24-hour urinary protein excretion estimation. The features described raise the suspicion of pre-eclampsia. A quantitative assay of the urinary protein excretion is essential to plan antenatal management.

Best of Fives (BOFs)

For the following statements choose the single best answer.

1. **With regards to tuberculosis in the UK, which of the following is true?**
   a) *Mycobacterium bovis* is responsible for 60% of cases of female genital tract infections.
   b) Involvement of the upper genital tract results from lymphatic spread of bacilli from a focus elsewhere in the body.
   c) Female genital tuberculosis may be sexually transmitted.
   d) HIV infection increases the risk of extrapulmonary disease.
   e) It is more common in postmenopausal women than in those in the reproductive age group.

2. **The main supports of the vagina include which of the following?**
   a) Iliopectineal ligaments
   b) Uterosacral ligaments
   c) Arcuate ligaments
   d) Round ligaments
   e) Obturator ligaments

3. **With regards to post-hysterectomy vaginal vault prolapse which of the following is true?**
   a) It can be successfully treated with a sacrocolpopexy.
   b) It is more common after abdominal hysterectomy.
   c) It is caused by excision of the uterosacral/round ligament complex.
   d) It can be successfully treated with a Burch colposuspension.
   e) It can be treated by a Manchester repair.

4. **With regards to amniocentesis which of the following is true?**
   a) If performed during the second trimester it leads to perforation of the placenta in up to 25% of cases.
   b) It carries a risk of severe sepsis in less than 1 in 2000 procedures.
   c) When compared with transcervical chorionic villous sampling, it has a 1% less miscarriage rate.
   d) When performed before 14 weeks of gestation, it is associated with up to 10 times the risk of fetal talipes.
   e) In the second trimester it carries no risk of transmission of HIV to the fetus.

5. A 25-year-old para 2 gravida 3 presents at 37 weeks gestation complaining of pain at the uterine fundus and fresh vaginal bleeding and is tender over the fundus of the uterus. Which of the following is most likely to be the diagnosis?
   a) Degenerating uterine fibroid.
   b) Pancreatitis.
   c) Placenta previa.
   d) Torted ovarian cyst.
   e) Placental abruption.

6. A para 2 gravida 2 has a normal delivery and, 8 days post-delivery, she complains of chest pain and shortness of breath. What is the most likely cause of her pain?
   a) Ruptured ovarian cyst.
   b) Amniotic fluid embolism.
   c) Pneumothorax.
   d) Pulmonary embolism.
   e) Pneumonia.

7. The ultrasound scan picture shows an exomphalos. Which of the following is not true?

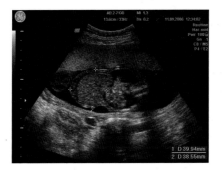

   a) Abdominal contents are contained within a sac.
   b) Liver herniates through the abdominal wall defect.
   c) The diagnosis is often associated with other congenital abnormalities.
   d) The mortality rate is 20%.
   e) It is also known as omphalocoele.

8. **A 55-year-old woman consults with you to discuss hormone replacement therapy. She has a strong family history of osteoporosis. Which is the most appropriate investigation?**
   a) MRI of spine and hip.
   b) Ultrasound densitometry of the wrist.
   c) Urinary markers of bone turnover.
   d) X-ray of spine and hip.
   e) Bone mineral density measurement or dual X-ray absorptiometry of spine and hip.

9. **A 50-year-old woman is found to have very low bone density, putting her at an increased risk of osteoporosis. Which of the following is not an appropriate single drug treatment for her?**
   a) Oestrogen replacement therapy.
   b) Progestogen replacement therapy.
   c) Strontium therapy.
   d) Tibolone.
   e) Raloxifene.

10. **In a normal pregnancy which of the following is true?**
    a) Arterial pCO_2 levels fall.
    b) Renal blood flow increases by 20%.
    c) Serum urea rises.
    d) Tidal volume decreases.
    e) Serum aldosterone decreases.

11. **With regards to endometrial cancer which of the following is true?**
    a) It is more common in women who are thin.
    b) The prognosis is better if vault irradiation is given preoperatively rather than postoperatively.
    c) PCOS is considered a risk factor.
    d) Histologically it is most commonly of squamous type.
    e) Initially it spreads to the inguinal nodes.

12. **Look at the figure shown. Which sentence best describes the photograph of the specimen?**

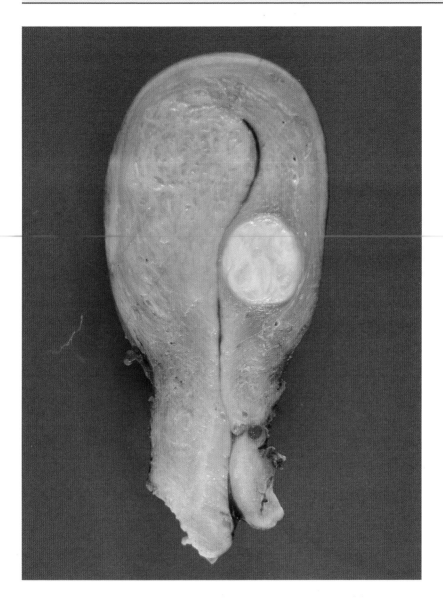

a) Adenomyosis in a uterus of normal size.
b) Intramural fibroid in a small uterus.
c) Subserous fibroid in an enlarged uterus.
d) Large submucous fibroid uterus.
e) Cervical polyp.

13. **With regards to chronic pelvic pain in women, which of the following is true?**
    a) The syndrome affects approximately 10% of women aged 18–50.
    b) Laparoscopic findings closely correlate with the severity of symptoms.
    c) Adhesiolysis is of proven benefit.
    d) Goserelin is an effective treatment.
    e) Laparoscopic uterine nerve ablation results in effective long-term symptom control (>1 year).

14. **Obstetric cholestasis is most prevalent in:**
    a) Ashkenazi Jews.
    b) Afro-Caribbeans.
    c) Asians.
    d) Araucanian Indians.
    e) Caucasians.

15. **A 17-year-old woman attends the genitourinary clinic with vaginal discharge and pelvic pain. Microscopy of an endocervical swab shows Gram-negative intracellular diplococci. She is allergic to penicillin. The most appropriate treatment is:**
    a) Intramuscular ceftriaxone 250 mg with oral probenecid 1 g orally.
    b) Intravenous ofloxacillin 400 mg b.d. + metronidazole 500 mg t.d.s. × 14 days.
    c) Oral ofloxacillin 400 mg b.d. + metronidazole 400 mg b.d. × 14 days.
    d) Intramuscular azithromycin 1 g + oral fusidic acid 500 mg t.d.s. × 14 days.
    e) Oral azithromycin 1 g daily × 14 days.

16. **With regards to endometrial ablation, which of the following is not true?**
    a) Amenorrhoea is not a usual consequence.
    b) Ideally the uterus is less than 12 weeks size.
    c) True dysmenorrhoea is significantly improved for most women.
    d) It provides contraception.
    e) Immediate risk of hysterectomy is about 1:2000.

17. **With regards to microwave endometrial ablation, which of the following is not true?**
    a) The technique is equally effective as an outpatient procedure or when performed under GA.
    b) The minimal uterine wall thickness should be 3 mm as detected by USS.

c) Depth of destruction is at least 5 mm from the contact surface.
d) Routine hysteroscopy should always precede MEA procedure.
e) It is designed to treat at temperature of 70–85°C.

18. Look at the figure shown. Which sentence best describes the photograph of the specimen?

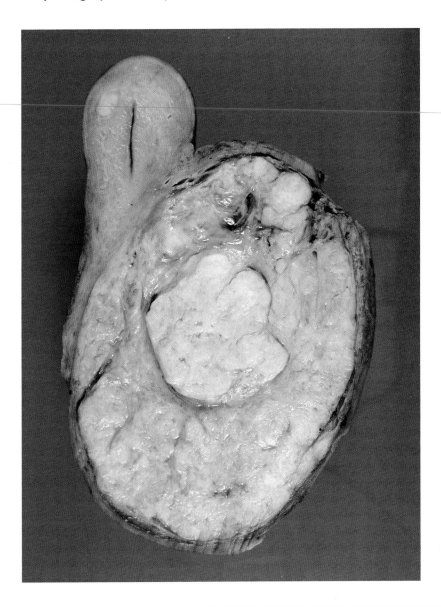

a) Cervical tumour in an enlarged uterus.
b) Large cervical fibroid and intramural fibroid in a small uterus.
c) Large cervical fibroid in a grossly enlarged uterus.
d) Cervical cancer.
e) Cervical polyp.

19. **The combined oral contraceptive pill is contraindicated in which of the following conditions?**
    a) Abnormal cervical smear under observation.
    b) History of unplanned pregnancy while taking combined OCP.
    c) Scanty or irregular periods.
    d) Past history of thrombosis.
    e) Severe depression.

20. **Which of the following is not an established risk factor for breast cancer?**
    a) Early menarche.
    b) High body mass index.
    c) Smoking.
    d) Age at birth of first child after 30 years.
    e) Use of combined HRT.

21. **Which of the following is least commonly associated with the Mirena IUS?**
    a) Pelvic inflammatory infection (post-insertion).
    b) Secondary amenorrhoea.
    c) Ectopic pregnancy.
    d) Irregular scanty bleeding.
    e) Improved dysmenorrhoea.

22. **With regards to cardiotocography, which of the following is not true?**
    a) The range of a normal fetal heart rate at term is 110–160 bpm.
    b) The baseline variability should range between 5 and 25 bpm.
    c) Fetal heart rate acceleration during a contraction is reassuring.
    d) Variable decelerations may be a sign of cord compression.
    e) An acceleration after a deceleration is a reassuring feature.

23. **The figure shows the ultrasound appearance of a double-bubble. What is the likely diagnosis?**

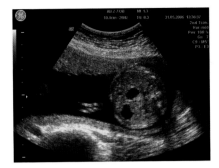

a) Pyloric stenosis.
b) Jejunal atresia.
c) Duodenal atresia.
d) Normal appearances.
e) Trisomy 13.

24. **With regards to trisomy, which of the following is true?**
    a) Trisomy 21 is usually the result of an error in maternal mitoses.
    b) Trisomy 21 occurs exclusively in women over 35 years of age.
    c) Trisomy 18 is often found in apparently normal children.
    d) PCR (polymerase chain reaction) is more cost effective than karyotyping for diagnosis.
    e) Trisomy 13 fetuses are often diagnosed by characteristic ultrasound features.

25. **With regards to Down's syndrome, which of the following is correct?**
    a) Marked differences in incidence between races have been shown.
    b) It causes no predisposition to malignancy.
    c) It may be associated with presenile dementia.
    d) Fetus has characteristic ultrasound diagnostic features.
    e) It is more common in male fetuses.

26. **Which of the following is not a feature of Turner's syndrome?**
    a) Short stature.
    b) Webbing of the fingers.
    c) Normal intelligence.
    d) Primary amenorrhoea.
    e) Increased risk of gonadoblastoma.

27. With regards to chicken pox in pregnancy which of the following is incorrect?

a) The disease is infectious from 48 hours before the rash appears until the vesicles crust over.

b) Oral acyclovir should be prescribed only within 24 hours of the onset of rash when pregnancy is more than 20 weeks gestation.

c) Varicella zoster immunoglobulin injection when given within 24 hours of contact prevents intrauterine infection and reduces the risk of fetal varicella syndrome.

d) Use of acyclovir in pregnancy is not associated with adverse fetal or neonatal effects.

e) Women who are known to be susceptible to varicella zoster virus infection should receive varicella zoster immunoglobulin injection as soon as possible after suspected exposure.

28. With regards to breech presentation, which of the following is incorrect?

a) The incidence is approximately 3% at term.

b) The recommended method of delivery of a term singleton breech is by planned caesarean section.

c) All women with an uncomplicated breech pregnancy at term should be offered external cephalic version.

d) Routine use of tocolysis is effective for external cephalic version.

e) The success rate of ECV is 75% in the UK.

29. Which of the following cardiotocographs best illustrates late decelerations?

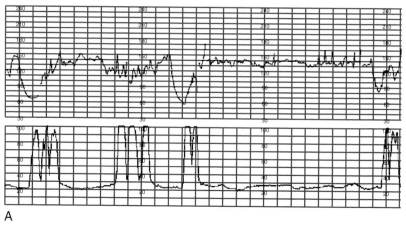

A

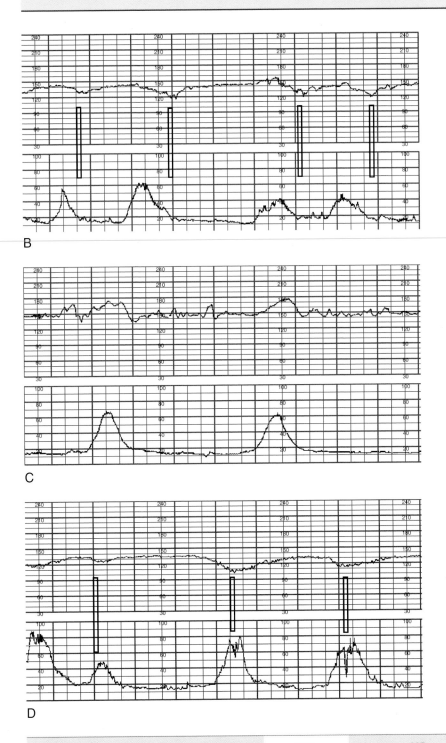

B

C

D

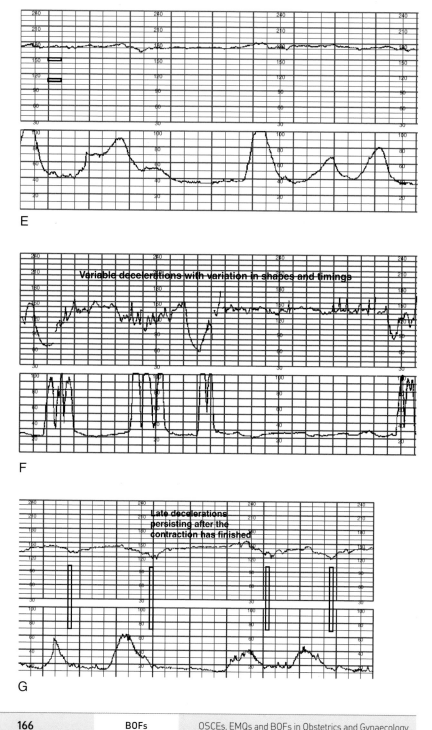

E

Variable decelerations with variation in shapes and timings

F

Late decelerations persisting after the contraction has finished

G

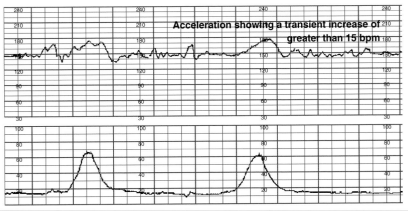

Acceleration showing a transient increase of greater than 15 bpm

H

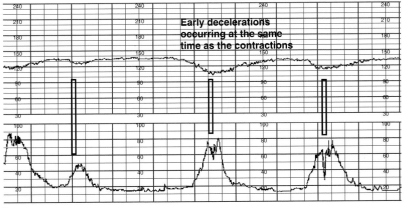

Early decelerations occurring at the same time as the contractions

I

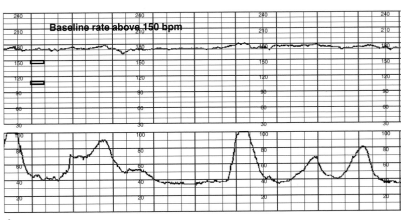

Baseline rate above 150 bpm

J

30. **With regards to tocolysis in preterm labour, which of the following is incorrect?**
    a) Atosiban is licensed and widely used.
    b) Nifedipine is not licensed for use in preterm labour.
    c) Maintenance therapy after cessation of contractions does not improve perinatal outcome.
    d) Magnesium sulphate is a recognised agent.
    e) Tocolytics should not be administered with steroids.

31. **Which of the following is not a risk factor for osteoporosis?**
    a) Premature ovarian failure.
    b) Diabetes.
    c) Afro-Caribbean origin.
    d) Smoking.
    e) Chronic liver disease.

32. **Which of the following is not a risk factor for pregnancy-induced hypertension?**
    a) Primigravida.
    b) Multiple pregnancy.
    c) Systemic lupus erythematosus.
    d) Smoking.
    e) Pregnancy with hydatidiform mole.

33. **With regards to metformin therapy in PCOS, which of the following is incorrect?**
    a) It improves the ovulation induction rate in clomifene citrate-resistant women with PCOS.
    b) It is associated with an increased risk of multiple pregnancy.
    c) It commonly causes hypoglycaemia in treated women with PCOS.
    d) It causes increased uptake of glucose by peripheral tissues.
    e) It is not licensed for use in PCOS.

34. **With regards to Down's syndrome, which of the following is incorrect?**
    a) It has a birth prevalence in the region of 1.4 per 1000 in England and Wales.
    b) It can be diagnosed using the triple test.

   c) It can be found in mosaic form.
   d) It is associated with polyhydramnios.
   e) It is associated with a higher rate of miscarriage than in pregnancies with a normal karyotype.

35. Which of the following is not known to be teratogenic?
   a) Alcohol.
   b) Methyldopa.
   c) Warfarin.
   d) Aminoglycosides.
   e) Phenytoin.

36. The following cytology slide is from a cervical smear. This shows:

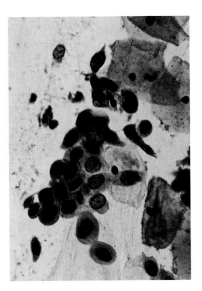

   a) Severe dyskaryosis.
   b) HPV.
   c) Normal cytology.
   d) Mild dyskaryosis.
   e) Moderate dyskaryosis.

37. **With regards to sickle cell disorders in pregnancy, which of the following is true?**
    a) Sickle cell disorders are most common in women of Asian origin.
    b) A sickle cell crisis can be precipitated in conditions of lowered oxygen tension.
    c) Sickle cell disorders are associated with an increased incidence of hypertension during pregnancy.
    d) Sickle cell disease results from a variant on the alpha globin chain.
    e) Partner screening is recommended during the second trimester.

38. **With regards to gonorrhoea, which of the following is incorrect?**
    a) It may cause blindness in the baby of an infected mother.
    b) It may cause perihepatitis.
    c) It may cause penile discharge.
    d) It is caused by a Gram-positive diplococcus.
    e) 50% of women are asymptomatic.

39. **In a pregnant woman whose first and only delivery was by lower segment caesarean section for a breech presentation, which of the following is true?**
    a) The chances of vaginal delivery are about 55%.
    b) The risk of scar rupture is over 1%.
    c) Erect lateral pelvimetry should be performed to exclude cephalopelvic disproportion.
    d) Intrauterine pressure monitoring has been shown to reduce the risk of uterine rupture.
    e) Continuous electronic fetal heart rate monitoring should be used in labour.

40. **With regards to puerperal psychosis, which of the following is true?**
    a) It occurs in about 1 in 1000 mothers.
    b) It is characteristically manic in type.
    c) It usually only results in a 2- to 3-week hospital stay.
    d) It is rarely recurrent.
    e) It is best treated by separation of the mother and the baby because of the risk of infanticide.

41. **Risks of combined oral contraceptive (COC) pill usage include (choose one):**
    a) Increased incidence of endometrial carcinoma.
    b) Pelvic inflammatory disease.
    c) Benign ovarian cysts.
    d) Hypotension.
    e) Decreased risk of ovarian carcinoma.

42. **This diagram illustrates what occurs during the normal menstrual cycle. 'Hormone A' is:**

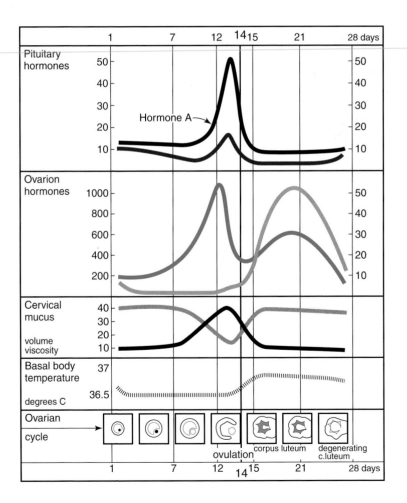

a) Oestrogen.
b) Progestogen.
c) Testosterone.
d) FSH.
e) LH.

43. **Congenital fetal malformations are not associated with the following maternal infections:**
    a) Syphilis.
    b) Toxoplasmosis.
    c) Cytomegalovirus.
    d) Measles.
    e) Parvovirus.

44. **With regards to a high fetal head at term in primipara, which of the following is incorrect?**
    a) It can be caused by placenta praevia.
    b) It can be caused by a lower segment uterine fibroid.
    c) It is associated with incorrect pregnancy dating.
    d) It is an indication for a caesarean section.
    e) It has a higher incidence in patients of African origin.

45. **With regards to LHRH analogues, which of the following is true?**
    a) They can be used to treat endometriosis.
    b) They rarely cause side-effects.
    c) They can be administered orally.
    d) They are inexpensive preparations.
    e) They act principally at the uterine level.

46. **With regards to the levonorgestrel IUS, which of the following is true?**
    a) It has been shown to increase endometrial hyperplasia.
    b) It has been shown to reduce endometriosis.
    c) It has been shown in randomised clinical trials to treat premenstrual syndrome.
    d) It can be used with oral oestrogen replacement therapy without the need for oral progestogen.
    e) It is associated with an increased rate of pelvic infection.

47. Which is the correct 10-year failure rate quoted for the method of sterilisation shown in the figure?

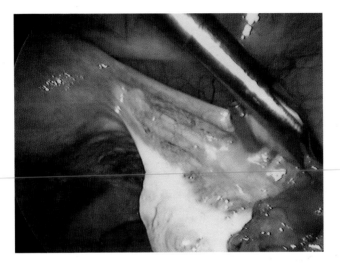

a) 1:500
b) 1:1000
c) 1:200
d) 1:300
e) 1:2000

48. With regards to anorexia nervosa, which of the following is incorrect?
a) It is associated with osteoporosis.
b) It has a 5–10% mortality.
c) Its sufferers have decreased skin collagen.
d) Amenorrhoea is the first sign to recover after treatment is started.
e) It is associated with a low FSH level.

49. With regards to *Candida albicans*, which of the following is true?
a) It is rarely asymptomatic.
b) Topical antifungals are more effective than oral antifungals.
c) Microscopy shows spores and pseudohyphae.
d) It has a recognised association with cervical dysplasia.
e) It has a recognised association with ovarian failure.

50. The causes of secondary amenorrhoea do not include:
a) Thyrotoxicosis.
b) Asherman's syndrome.
c) Endometriosis.
d) Premature ovarian failure.
e) Virilising ovarian tumour.

51. The following is a drawing of the fetal skull diameters. The diameter highlighted in red is the:

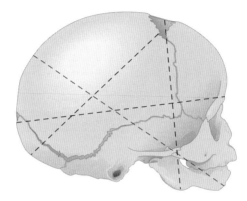

a) Occipitofrontal.
b) Suboccipitobregmatic.
c) Mentovertical.
d) Subabregmatic.
e) Biparietal.

52. With regards to the fetal skull, which of the following is incorrect?
a) The biparietal diameter is approximately 9.5 cm at term.
b) The lambdoidal suture runs between the parietal, temporal and occipital bones.
c) The bregma is the area lying between the parietal and occipital bones.
d) The suboccipital bregmatic diameter is the engaging diameter when the head is fully flexed in a vertex presentation.
e) The chin is the denominator in a face presentation.

53. **With regards to the progesterone-only pill, which of the following is true?**
    a) It increases tubal mobility.
    b) It acts mainly by inhibiting ovulation.
    c) It should not be prescribed to someone who has a history of a deep vein thrombosis.
    d) It can be safely given to lactating women.
    e) It does not cause amenorrhoea.

54. **With regards to precocious puberty, which of the following is incorrect?**
    a) Breast buds are the first sign.
    b) It is usually constitutional.
    c) It is associated with long bone fractures.
    d) It results in tall stature.
    e) It can be halted by GNRH analogues.

55. **With regards to trisomy 18, which of the following is incorrect?**
    a) 50% die by 2 months.
    b) It is age related.
    c) Choroid plexus cysts are often present.
    d) They are commonly delivered by caesarean section for fetal distress.
    e) They are always female.

56. **With regards to group B streptococcal colonisation in pregnancy, which of the following is false?**
    a) It is present in approximately 25–30% of the pregnant population.
    b) Group B Streptococci are facultative, anaerobic, gm +ve bacteria.
    c) The rate of colonisation varies between different ethnic groups.
    d) The colonisation is chronic rather than transient or intermittent.
    e) The colonisation is usually asymptomatic.

57. **With regards to hyperemesis gravidarum (HG) which of the following is false?**
    a) It affects about 1% of pregnancies.
    b) Diagnosis is based on maternal weight loss of over 5% body mass and ketosis.
    c) It is more common among women with a past history of eating disorder.

d) All women should receive vitamin B_1 supplement.

e) Biochemical evidence of hyperthyroidism should trigger early treatment.

58. Oligohydramnios is associated with all of the following except:

a) Renal agenesis.

b) Twin-twin transfusion syndrome in monochorionic twin pregnancies.

c) Talipes in the infant.

d) Pulmonary hypoplasia.

e) Oesophageal atresia.

59. This is the sagittal section of a female pelvis, illustrating the types of prolapse that can occur. The arrow 'B' represents:

a) Rectocele.

b) Uterine prolapse.

c) Enterocele.

d) Urethrocele.

e) Cystocele.

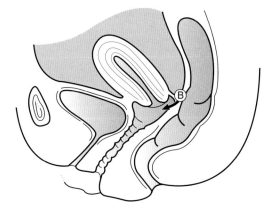

60. Non-surgical interventions for urinary stress incontinence include all except:

a) Pelvic floor physiotherapy.

b) Weight loss.

c) Venlafaxine.

d) Bladder neck support devices.

e) Cessation of smoking.

1. c) **Female genital tuberculosis may be sexually transmitted**
       Pelvic inflammatory disease may be associated with
       mycobacterium tuberculosis due to dissemination of the
       microorganism via the bloodstream. Primary infection of the
       vulva, vagina and cervix may result from direct inoculation at
       sexual intercourse with persons having genitourinary tuberculosis.

2. b) **Uterosacral ligaments**
       The uterosacral ligament is fibromuscular and passes from the
       pericervical ring to the sacrum. It supports the cervix and apex of
       the vagina.

3. a) **It can be successfully be treated with a sacrocolpopexy**
       In cases of recurrent vault prolapse, most surgeons would prefer
       the abdominal route and perform a sacrocolpopexy. In this
       procedure the vaginal vault is attached by a mesh to the anterior
       longitudinal ligament over the first or second sacral vertebra.

4. d) **When performed before 14 weeks of gestation,
       is associated with up to 10 times the risk of fetal talipes**
       Amniocentesis is ideally performed between 15 and 18 weeks
       and the risk of pregnancy loss after the procedure is 1% higher
       than the background loss rate at any given gestation.

5. e) **Placental abruption**
       In any woman presenting in the third trimester with abdominal
       pain, tender uterus and bleeding, placental abruption must be
       excluded.

6. d) **Pulmonary embolism**
       Thromboembolic disease is an important cause of maternal
       mortality and the risk during pregnancy and in the puerperium is
       six times higher than in the non-pregnant state.

7. d) **The mortality rate is 20%.**
       Mortality rates from exomphalos are quoted at 5–10%.

8. e) **Bone mineral density measurement or dual X-ray
       absorptiometry of spine and hip**
       Dual energy X-ray absorptiometry is currently the most available,
       accurate tool for measuring bone density.

9. b) Progestogen replacement therapy

Progestogen replacement therapy will provide some protection against bone loss, but not enough for someone who is at increased risk of osteoporosis.

10. a) Arterial pCO_2 levels fall

Respiratory rate remains constant during pregnancy, whereas tidal volume increases, therefore the minute ventilation also increases. As a result of this, and the effect of progesterone increasing the level of carbonic anhydrase B in red cells, arterial pCO_2 falls in pregnancy. At the same time, there is a fall in plasma bicarbonate concentration and the arterial pH therefore remains constant.

11. c) PCOS is considered a risk factor

In PCOS the LH/FSH ratio and serum oestradiol are raised. The high oestrogen levels may lead to hyperplastic changes to the endometrium which, in turn, can lead to malignant change.

12. d) Large submucous fibroid uterus

The uterus itself is enlarged (approximately 12×6 cm^2) with a large submucous fibroid (approximately 2 cm diameter).

13. d) Goserelin is an effective treatment

Ovarian suppression may be an effective treatment for pain associated with endometriosis. This may be achieved with a gonadotrophin releasing hormone agonist such as goserelin. Goserelin has been shown to be effective in small RCTs.

14. d) Araucanian Indians

Obstetric cholestasis demonstrates a racial distribution. In the UK it affects 0.7% of pregnancies and the prevalence is approximately double in women of Indian/Pakistani Asian origin. The highest prevalence is documented in Chile.

15. c) Oral ofloxacillin 400 mg b.d. + metronidazole 400 mg b.d. × 14 days

The diagnosis is gonococcal infection and the usual treatment is penicillin. As there is an allergy to penicillin the appropriate alternative is ofloxacillin. Metronidazole is added to treat the common co-existing infection with anaerobic organisms.

16. d) It provides contraception

Endometrial ablation is not a method of contraception and alternative methods should be advised. Pregnancy is unlikely but has been reported.

17. b) The minimal uterine wall thickness should be 3 mm as detected by USS

The information produced by the manufacturers of MEA states that ultrasound scan determined thickness of the uterine myometrium should be at least 10 mm before MEA is considered safe.

18. b) Large cervical fibroid and intramural fibroid in a small uterus

The photograph shows the typical cross-sectional appearance of a large fibroid arising in the cervix. The uterus itself is small with a much smaller intramural fibroid.

19. d) Past history of thrombosis

Past history of venous or arterial thrombosis is an absolute contraindication to the combined oral contraceptive pill.

20. c) Smoking

Most studies have not shown a link between smoking and breast cancer risk.

21. c) Ectopic pregnancy

The ectopic pregnancy rate for the levonorgestrel releasing IUS is quoted as 0.02 per 100 woman years.

22. e) An acceleration after a deceleration is a reassuring feature

An acceleration after a deceleration implies hypoxia ± acidaemia during the deceleration resulting in a transient compensatory fetal tachycardia.

23. c) Duodenal atresia

A double bubble sign seen on cross-sectional ultrasound scan of the fetal abdomen is indicative of duodenal atresia.
Jejunal atresia usually gives rise to a triple bubble.

24. d) PCR (polymerase chain reaction) is more cost effective than karyotyping for diagnosis

The technique of fluorescent polymerase chain reaction is a rapid and inexpensive method for prenatal diagnosis of trisomy 21.

25. c) It may be associated with presenile dementia

Alzheimer's is commoner in Down's syndrome than in the overall population.

26. b) Webbing of the fingers

Turner's syndrome is associated with webbing of the neck.

27. c) Varicella zoster immunoglobulin injection when given within 24 hours of contact prevents intrauterine infection and reduces the risk of fetal varicella syndrome

There is no evidence that administration of varicella zoster immunoglobulin within 24 hours of contact with chickenpox prevents intrauterine infection.

28. e) The success rate of ECV is 75% in the UK

The success rate of external cephalic version at term, from studies in the UK, is less than 50%.

29. b)

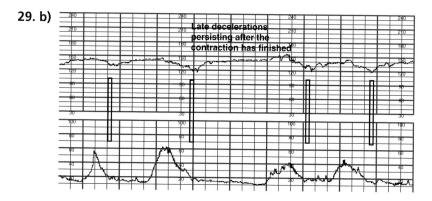

30. e) Tocolytics should not be administered with steroids

One of the main indications for tocolysis in preterm labour is to administer betamethasone. In diabetic mothers the combination should only be used with an insulin sliding scale regimen.

31. c) Afro-Caribbean origin

Afro-Caribbean women have a bone mineral density higher than that of white women at all ages. White women have a 2.5-fold greater risk of osteoporosis.

32. d) Smoking

Smoking in pregnancy does not appear to be associated with increased risk of pre-eclampsia.

33. c) It commonly causes hypoglycaemia in treated women with PCOS

The most common side-effects of metformin therapy are gastrointestinal. Hypoglycaemia does not usually occur.

34. b) It can be diagnosed using the triple test

The triple test uses serum markers combined with the age of the mother and confirmed gestation of the pregnancy to give a calculated estimate of risk of Down's syndrome. The screening test is not diagnostic.

35. b) Methyldopa

Methyldopa has now been used for many years for hypertension in pregnancy and is not known to be teratogenic.

36. a) Severe dyskaryosis

Dyskaryosis cells are recognisable as a squamous cell, but display some of the features of malignancy: the nucleus is enlarged, the chromatin is increased and the nuclear borders are irregular.

37. b) A sickle cell crisis can be precipitated in conditions of lowered oxygen tension

The rates of miscarriage, pre-term labour and fetal loss are increased in women who have sickle cell disorders.

38. d) It is caused by a Gram-positive diplococcus

Gonorrhoea is caused by a Gram-negative diplococcus.

39. e) Continuous electronic fetal heart rate monitoring should be used in labour

Approximately 70% of women with one previous caesarean section will achieve a vaginal delivery. Rupture of the uterine scar can occur in up to 0.5% of these women, so a 'trial of labour' must be carefully managed. Intrapartum care must include continuous electronic fetal heart rate monitoring.

40. a) It occurs in about 1 in 1000 mothers

Psychosis is rare and is usually depressive in nature. Risk factors are: previous post-partum psychiatric disorder, previous psychiatric history, previous still birth or early neonatal death, ambivalence about motherhood or relationship with her partner, lack of social contacts and a major problem in the pregnancy or puerperium.

41. e) Decreased risk of ovarian carcinoma

If the oral contraceptive pill is taken for more than 5 years, there is a 50% reduction in ovarian cancer and 40% reduction in endometrial cancer.

42. e) LH

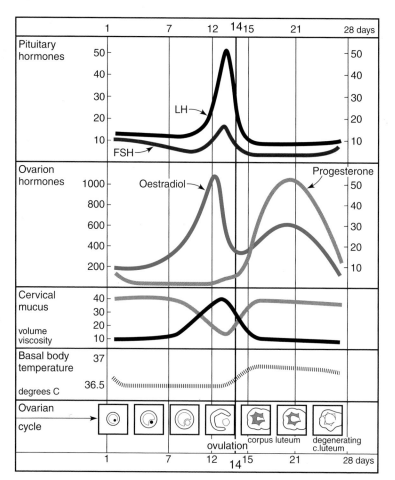

The diagram shows the pituitary, ovarian and endometrial changes during the menstrual cycle.

43. d) Measles

Congenital fetal malformations are associated with chicken pox, rubella, syphilis, toxoplasmosis, CMV and parvovirus.

44. d) It is an indication for a caesarean section

A high fetal head at term in a primiparous patient is, in itself, not an indication for abdominal delivery as 10% will not engage until labour commences.

45. a) They can be used to treat endometriosis

Leutinising hormone releasing hormone analogues are administered by injection, implant or nasally and induce a temporary menopause. They initially stimulate (partial agonist activity) but subsequently cause down-regulation of receptors at the pituitary gland.

46. d) It can be used with oral oestrogen replacement therapy without the need for oral progestogen

The levonorgestrel IUS is used for pelvic endometriosis but there are, as yet, no data to confirm efficacy.

47. c) 1:200

The photograph shows laparoscopic application of a Filshie clip to the isthmic portion of the right fallopian tube. The accepted long-term pregnancy rate for this method of sterilisation is 1:200.

48. d) Amenorrhoea is the first sign to recover after treatment is started

Weight gain is the first sign of recovery after treatment of anorexia nervosa. Some women remain amenorrhoeic despite weight gain.

49. c) Microscopy shows spores and pseudohyphae

Candida albicans is a very common cause of abnormal vaginal discharge, occurring at any age. Ten of 20% to women of reproductive age have asymptomatic Candida.

50. c) Endometriosis

The aetiology of secondary amenorrhoea can broadly be divided into five compartments: target organ and outflow tract dysfunction, gonadal failure, pituitary dysfunction, hypothalamic dysfunction, thyroid or adrenal dysfunction.

51. c) Mentovertical

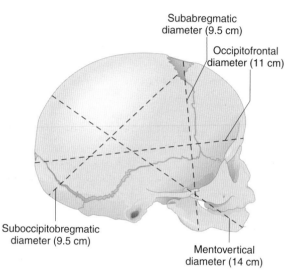

Subabregmatic diameter (9.5 cm)

Occipitofrontal diameter (11 cm)

Suboccipitobregmatic diameter (9.5 cm)

Mentovertical diameter (14 cm)

52. c) The bregma is the area lying between the parietal and occipital bones

The bregma (anterior fontanelle) is the large, diamond-shaped depression where the frontal, coronal and sagittal sutures meet.

53. d) It can be safely given to lactating women

The progesterone-only pill (POP) thickens the cervical mucus to inhibit sperm entry through the cervical canal. The POP also thins the endometrium and, in some women, inhibits ovulation.

54. d) It results in tall stature

Precocious onset of puberty is defined as occurring younger than 2 standard deviations before the average age, that is, less than 8 years old in females. Thus, in many girls, early onset of puberty merely represents one end of the normal distribution. It is important to exclude pathological causes such as congenital adrenal hyperplasia, cranial or peripheral tumours. Continuous, high levels of a gonadotrophin releasing hormone analogue may be used to inhibit puberty. The aims of stopping puberty are to avoid psychosocial problems arising from early sexual maturation and to prevent reduction in final adult height due to premature bone maturation and early epiphyseal fusion.

55. e) They are always female
Trisomy 18 is Edward's syndrome and is usually associated with multiple congenital abnormalities and death in the newborn period.

56. d) The colonisation is chronic rather than transient or intermittent
Colonisation of the female genital tract occurs in an intermittent manner.

57. e) Biochemical evidence of hyperthyroidism should trigger early treatment
Biochemical evidence of hyperthyroidism is common (approximately 60% of women with hyperemesis gravidarum) and self-limiting.

58. e) Oesophageal atresia
Oesophageal atresia is associated with polyhydramnios.

59. c) Enterocele

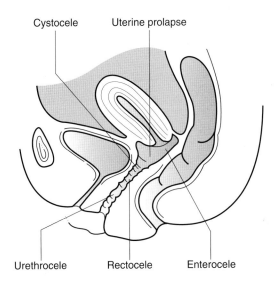

60. c) Venlafaxine

The serotonin and noradrenaline reuptake inhibitor duloxetine is a licensed treatment for urinary stress incontinence.